IMMUNOTHERAPY:
Cellular Transplants &
Immunostimulation

Papers by
E. Richard Stiehm, Dale E. Bockman,
D. Amato et al.

MSS Information Corporation
655 Madison Avenue, New York, N.Y. 10021

Library of Congress Cataloging in Publication Data
Main entry under title:

Immunotherapy: current research.

CONTENTS: Stiehm, E. R., and others. Immunologic
reconstitution in severe combined immunodeficiency without bone-marrow chromosomal chemerism.--Bockman, D. E.,
Lawton, A. R., and Cooper, M. D. Fine structure of
thymus after bone marrow transplantation in an infant
with severe combined immunodeficiency.--Amato, D., and
others. Review of bone marrow transplants at the
Ontario Cancer Institute. [etc.]
1. Immunotherapy--Addresses, essays, lectures.
I. Stiehm, E. Richard, 1933-   [DNLM: 1. Bone
marrow cells--Transplantation--Collected Works.
2. Immunotherapy--Collected Works. QW504 I363 1974]

RM275.I48   615'.36   74-591
ISBN 0-8422-7199-6

TABLE OF CONTENTS

CREDITS AND ACKNOWLEDGEMENTS

Amato, D.; D.E. Bergsagel; A.M. Clarysse; D.H. Cowan; N.N. Iscove; E.A. McCulloch; R.G. Miller; R.A. Phillips; A.H. Ragab; and J.S. Senn, "Review of Bone Marrow Transplants at the Ontario Cancer Institute," *Transplantation Proceedings*, 1971, 3:397-399.

Ammann, A.J.; H.J. Meuwissen; R.A. Good; and R. Hong, "Successful Bone Marrow Transplantation in a Patient with Humoral and Cellular Immunity Deficiency," *Clinical and Experimental Immunology*, 1970, 7:343-353.

Ammann, Arthur J.; Diane W. Wara; Sydney Salmon; and Herbert Perkins, "Thymus Transplantation. Permanent Reconstitution of Cellular Immunity in a Patient with Sex-Linked Combined Immunodeficiency," *New England Journal of Medicine*, 1973, 289:5-9.

Bockman, Dale E.; Alexander R. Lawton; and Max D. Cooper, "Fine Structure of Thymus after Bone Marrow Transplantation in an Infant with Severe Combined Immunodeficiency," *Laboratory Investigation*, 1972, 26:227-239.

Buckner, C.D.; R.A. Clift; A. Fefer; D.D. Funk; H. Glucksberg; R.E. Ramberg; R. Storb; and E.D. Thomas, "Aplastic Anemia Treated by Marrow Transplantation," *Transplantation Proceedings*, 1973, 5:913-916.

Dicke, K.A.; U.W. Schaefer; and D.W. van Bekkum, "The Use of Stem Cell Concentrates as Bone Marrow Grafts in Man," *Transplantation Proceedings*, 1973, 5:909-912.

Fefer, A.; C.D. Buckner; R.A. Clift; L. Fass; K.G. Lerner; E.M. Mickelson; P. Neiman; R. Rudolph; R. Storb; and E.D. Thomas, "Marrow Grafting in Identical Twins with Hematologic Malignancies," *Transplantation Proceedings*, 1973, 5:927-931.

Hanna, M.G. Jr.; M.J. Snodgrass; Berton Zbar; and Herbert J. Rapp, "Histopathology of *Mycobacterium bovis* (BCG)-Mediated Tumor Regression," *National Cancer Institute Monograph No. 35*, pp. 345-357.

Katz, David H.; Leonard Ellman; William E. Paul; Ira Green; and Baruj Benacerraf, "Resistance of Guinea Pigs to Leukemia following Transfer of Immunocompetent Allogeneic Lymphoid Cells," *Cancer Research*, 1972, 32:133-140.

Kirkpatrick, C.H.; R.R. Rich; R.G. Graw, Jr.; T.K. Smith; Irad; Mickenberg; and G.N. Rogentine, "Treatment of Chronic Mucocutaneous Moniliasis by Immunologic Reconstitution," *Clinical and Experimental Immunology*, 1971, 9:733-748.

Marcolongo, Roberto; and Nicola Di Paolo, "Fetal Thymic Transplant in Patients with Hodgkin's Disease," *Blood*, 1973, 41:625-633.

Marshall, W.H., "Transfer of Immune Responsiveness," *Medical Clinics of North America*, 1972, 56:465-480.

Mitchison, N.A., "Immunologic Approach to Cancer," *Transplantation Proceedings*, 1970, 2:92-103.

Santos, George W., "Application of Marrow Grafts in Human Disease," *American Journal of Pathology*, 1971, 65:653-668.

Stiehm, E. Richard; Glenn J. Lawlor, Jr.; Michael S. Kaplan; Harris L. Greenwald; Robert C. Neerhout; Dharmendra P.S. Sengar; and Paul I. Terasaki, "Immunologic Reconstitution in Severe Combined Immunodeficiency without Bone-Marrow Chromosomal Chimerism," *New England Journal of Medicine*, 1972, 286:797-803.

PREFACE

The transfer of immune responsiveness from one individual within a species to another was first demonstrated more than thirty years ago. Initially this transfer was effected with live lymphoid cells. Although the finding was subsequently repeated in a variety of species, including man, the technique was of limited therapeutic use for two reasons. The major problem was that the transferred lymphocytes, immunologically competent in their own right, often responded to the tissue of the host, giving rise to a "graft-versus-host" response, GVH. The consequence of the GVH was often fatal. Secondly, the transplanted lymphocytes often also evoked a response from the host, resulting in the destruction or rejection of the grafted cells. Thus, any benefit from the grafted lymphocytes was short lived. Through more knowledge of the immune mechanism as well as the histocompatibility antigen system of man, it later became clear that the former problems connected with immunotherapy could be solved. Further more, H.S. Lawrence made the discovery in 1954 that certain types of immune reactivity could be transferred from one human to another using a soluble extract of lymphocytes. This substance, now known as "transfer factor," laid the ground work for an effective approach to immunotherapy without the early problems one faced with whole cells.

Since these early findings, immunologists have greatly advanced their conceptual understanding of manipulating the immune response in man. The clinician can now boost or prime one's immune system to better ward off infectious disease and malignant cells that may arise. Through an appreciation of the defects in immunodeficiency disease, it is also possible for an effected individual to be reconstituted with populations of stem cells which can develop to mature lymphocytes. Most encouraging is the general belief that these therapeutic achievements signal a new era in medicine, and as our understanding of immunity becomes clearer, so will the means of effective manipulation.

This first in a two volume series on Immunotherapy presents literature concerned with the transfer of immune responsiveness via whole cells. Section I deals with a number of clinical studies in which bone marrow transplants have been utilized in the treatment of humans. There are also other procedures such as thymic and lymphocyte grafts which are being used with increasing success. Perhaps the most exciting and controversial immunotherapeutic approach is that used in treating malignancies. Here an affected individual is given various forms of immunostimulants in an attempt to directly or indirectly provoke the immune mechanism to destroy the tumor. This latter treatment regimen shows potential but has not appeared as promising as the former approaches. However, these topics are covered in Section II, and the literature provides an up to date survey of the "state of the art." There are still hazards which must be overcome but the potential for new forms of therapy outweigh the shortcomings and serve as a stimulus for new research.

Ronald T. Acton, Ph.D.
March, 1974

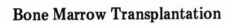

Bone Marrow Transplantation

IMMUNOLOGIC RECONSTITUTION IN SEVERE COMBINED IMMUNODEFICIENCY WITHOUT BONE-MARROW CHROMOSOMAL CHIMERISM

E. RICHARD STIEHM, M.D., GLENN J. LAWLOR, JR., M.D.,

MICHAEL S. KAPLAN, M.D., HARRIS L. GREENWALD, M.D.,

ROBERT C. NEERHOUT, M.D., DHARMENDRA P.S. SENGAR, PH.D.,

AND PAUL I. TERASAKI, PH.D.

Abstract An 11-month-old male infant with severe combined immunodeficiency was immunologically reconstituted by bone-marrow transplantation from a female sibling whose cells were HL-A compatible on mixed leukocyte culture. The patient's lymphocytes demonstrated multiple extraneous HL-A antigens (up to 10 at one time), some of which were not present in the parents or the four siblings; this typing anomaly delayed bone-marrow donor selection. These additional antigens were nonstimulatory in mixed leukocyte culture, and since they were found in two similar patients, may represent an anomaly peculiar to combined immunodeficiency.

After leukocyte transfer factor was given without benefit on two occasions, bone-marrow transplantation was performed. After a severe graft-versus-host reaction subsided, clinical improvement and chimerism ensued as evidenced by an XX (donor) karyotype of cultured peripheral blood lymphocytes and restoration of immunologic functions. Direct chromosome analysis of bone-marrow cells disclosed only XY cells, despite the presence of plasma cells synthesizing IgG-globulin of the donor's genetic type.

BONE-marrow transplantation in severe combined immunodeficiency* (Swiss-type agammaglobulinemia) from an HL-A identical sibling may reverse a disorder characterized by a progressive downhill course with death, usually by one year of age. Since 1968, when Gatti and his associates reported the first successful bone-marrow transplantation in this disorder,[2] at least 16 other patients have received transplants,[3] most of which have demon-

Supported in part by research grants (ES 00391, AM 02375, AI 04444, and AM 07513) and general research-support funds from the National Institutes of Health.

*Nomenclature recommended by a World Health Organization committee on primary immunodeficiencies.[1]

11

strated engraftment as determined by chromosomal chimerism. Three of these patients are surviving for over three years.[4-7] Although the cellular immunodeficiency permits successful engraftment, varying degrees of graft-versus-host (GVH) reactions have developed in all these patients, presumably because of minor histocompatibility antigen differences. These GVH reactions are nonfatal and self-limited; in contrast, the GVH reaction has proved to be fatal in all cases when HL-A differences exist.[8]

We recently treated a male infant with several of the characteristics of severe combined immunodeficiency, including profound humoral and cellular immunodeficiencies, *Pneumocystis carinii* pneumonia, oral and esophageal moniliasis and a progressive downhill course. Repeated examination of the patient's lymphocytes disclosed multiple (up to 10) extraneous HL-A types, some of which were not found in the parents and four siblings. Bone-marrow transplantation from the patient's sister was performed at the age of 11 months. After the patient survived a severe GVH reaction, there was dramatic clinical improvement and laboratory evidence of chimerism and immunologic reconstitution; however, the bone marrow gives no evidence of chromosomal chimerism.

CASE REPORT

A male infant was the product of a normal term pregnancy and delivery; the birth weight was 3200 g. The neonatal period was unremarkable except for persistent rhinorrhea. He received 2 diphtheria-pertussis-tetanus and oral poliomyelitis immunizations at the ages of 3 and 4 months. At 3½ months, thrush that did not respond to mycostatin developed. Ten days later, fever, respiratory difficulty, cough and anorexia occurred; erythromycin was given, without benefit. He was admitted to the UCLA Medical Center at 5 months of age.

The mother, the father, a brother and 3 sisters were well. There was no consanguinity. Three maternal male cousins had cystic fibrosis; 2 had died in infancy. One maternal male cousin had died at the age of 5 days with leukopenia. The family lived in a semirural area with numerous pets, including dogs, cats, horses and rabbits.

Physical examination revealed a mildly ill infant with a few rales in the chest and oral moniliasis. The weight was 7.0 kg. No tonsillar tissue or adenopathy was present. The white-cell count was 10,000, with 50 per cent neutrophils and 35 per cent lymphocytes. Chest x-ray study revealed bilateral infiltrates. Ampicillin was given, with clinical improvement, and the patient was discharged after 5 days with immunologic studies pending. He was readmitted to the hospital 3 days later with recurrent fever, increased respiratory distress and persistent thrush. The temperature was 37.4°C, the

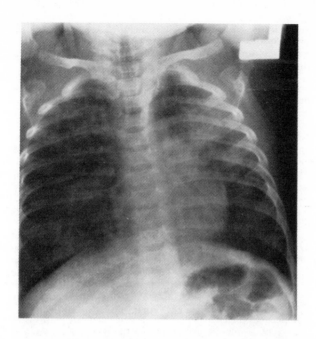

Figure 1. Roentgenogram of the Chest at the Age of Six Months, Showing Pneumonia with Extensive Peribronchial Disease, a Confluent Infiltrate in the Left Upper Lobe and Multiple Small Cystic Areas of Uninvolved Lung between the Areas of Cystic Disease.

P. carinii organisms were demonstrated by needle aspirate. No thymic shadow is present.

pulse 140, and the respirations 44. He was in moderate respiratory distress, with moist rales at both lung bases.

The hemoglobin was 12.9 g per 100 ml, the hematocrit 36 per cent, and the white-cell count 22,400, with 59 per cent neutrophils, 33 per cent lymphocytes, 4 per cent eosinophils and 4 per cent monocytes. Both small and large lymphocytes of normal morphology were present on the peripheral blood smear. The erythrocyte sedimentation rate (Wintrobe method) was 4 mm per hour. A bone-marrow aspirate was normal; however, no plasma cells were present. Total serum immunoglobulins were 150 mg per 100 ml. Skin tests to 5 U of purified protein derivative (PPD), 1:10 dermatophytin (monilia), 100 U of streptokinase and 25 U of streptodornase (SK-SD), mumps skin-test antigen, 1:10 trichophyton and 0.1 mg of dinitrofluorobenzene (after a sensitizing application) were negative. A Schick test was reactive (positive), and isoagglutinins and poliomyelitis neutralization antibodies were negative. The blood was type O, Rh negative. Peripheral lymphocytes cultured with phytohemagglutinin (PHA) or mitomycin-treated allogeneic cells did not proliferate (Table 1). A diagnosis of severe combined immunodeficiency was made.

Repeat x-ray examination revealed progression of the pulmonary infiltrate (Fig. 1). Respiratory distress became more severe, despite ampicillin therapy. A needle lung aspirate disclosed *P. carinii* organisms. Pentamidine isethionate was given for 2 weeks (total dose, 392 mg), during which there was gradual improvement.

The patient's lymphocytes were HL-A typed on several occasions; because of the presence of multiple antigens not present in either parent and an apparent lymphocyte type not identical to any sibling, bone-marrow transplantation was postponed.

Biweekly gamma-globulin injections and gentian-violet applications to the mouth were begun. Over the next 3 months there were intermittent fevers, poor feeding and no weight gain (Fig. 2). In an effort to control the oral moniliasis by restoration of specific cellular immunity,[9] leukocyte transfer factor from monilia-positive subjects was given on 2 separate occasions. There was no clinical improvement, and the monilia skin test remained negative.

The patient was readmitted to the hospital at 9 months of age because of vomiting and weight loss. Barium esophagraphy was compatible with extensive monilial esophagitis (Fig. 3). A 5-week course of intravenous amphotericin (total dose of 127 mg) and nasogastric-tube feedings resulted in resolution of the esophagitis, but the oral moniliasis remitted only temporarily.

Repeat lymphocyte typing and mixed leukocyte cultures at the age of 11 months disclosed that the patient's 12-year-old sister was apparently HL-A compatible by mixed leukocyte culture. The sister was type O, Rh positive, had a positive skin test to monilia, had normal immunoglobulins, and had lymphocytes that were normally reactive in vitro to phytohemagglutinin and allogeneic cells (Table 1).

Bone-marrow transplantation was performed on February 3, 1971. Under general anesthesia, 150 ml of marrow was aspirated from multiple sternal and iliac-crest sites from the 12-year-old sister. The marrow was heparinized, mixed with

Table 1. Mixed-Leukocyte-Culture Response of the Patient and the Sibling Donor.*

RESPONDING CELLS	HL-A TYPES	STIMULATING CELLS (MITOMYCIN TREATED)†			
		Am	Bm	Cm	Dm
A. Patient	HL-A2,Te52/ HL-A2,Te54 (haplotypes)	163	212 (1.30)	204 (1.25)	192 (1.17)
B. Sibling donor	HL-A2,Te52/ HL-A2,Te54 (haplotypes)	209 (1.43)	146	2640 (18.08)	3192 (21.86)
C. Unrelated control	HL-A2, HL-A5, Te40 (phenotype)	8543 (13.35)	4982 (7.78)	640	3301 (5.16)
D. Unrelated control	HL-A3,HL-A9, HL-A5,Te60 (phenotype)	7798 (11.12)	6499 (9.27)	‡	701

*All tests were done with 0.05 × 10⁶ responding & an equal no. of stimulating cells in triplicates.
†Figures in parentheses refer to ratio of cpm in stimulated vs control cultures; ratios >2.3 are statistically significant.
‡Not done.

14

TC-199 tissue culture medium and placed in a blood-donor bag; 80 ml containing 2 × 10⁹ nucleated marrow cells was given intraperitoneally to the patient, without complications.

Two weeks after transplantation, a positive skin test to monilia (1:10) developed, and the oral moniliasis disappeared. Isoagglutinins became detectable 2½ weeks after transplantation, and the serum immunoglobulins began to increase 4½ weeks after transplantation (Fig. 2). Six weeks after transplantation the peripheral lymphocytes became reactive to phytohemagglutinin and demonstrated an XX (donor) karyotype. Bone-marrow examination disclosed plasma cells.

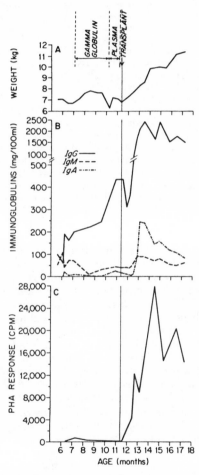

Figure 2. Course of the Patient before and after Marrow Transplantation at the Age of 11 Months, Showing the Weight in Kilograms (Top), IgG, IgM and IgA Immunoglobulins in Milligrams per 100 Ml (Middle) and in Vitro Lymphocyte Response to Phytohemagglutinin (PHA) as Assayed by Incorporation of ³H-Thymidine and Expressed in Counts per Minute (Bottom).

15

Eighteen days after transplantation, a maculopapular rash over the face and trunk developed that became generalized and desquamative. Three days later, a temperature of 39.2°C, submandibular adenopathy, hepatosplenomegaly, conjunctivitis and respiratory distress, with cyanosis, tachypnea and tachycardia, occurred. X-ray study disclosed an infiltrate in the right hilar area (Fig. 4). The white-cell count was 15,000, with 10 per cent lymphocytes. The platelets, eosinophils and reticulocytes remained unchanged. A Coombs test was negative. An electrocardiogram was normal, and a lung aspirate showed no *P. carinii* organisms or other pathogens. The patient was placed in a sterile environment and given oxygen, intravenous fluids, mafenide acetate (Sulfamylon) cream to the skin, digoxin and 2 5-ml injections of pseudomonas immune globulin (human). He was also given a single dose of prednisone (5 mg), but since improvement had begun, this therapy was not continued. The apparent graft-versus-host reaction gradually subsided after 10 days, but hepatosplenomegaly and the chest infiltrate persisted. He was discharged from the hospital 52 days after transplantation.

Since discharge he has done well and at the age of 21 months was in the 50th percentile for height and weight. Three months after transplantation, fever, rhinorrhea and a maculopapular rash on the scalp and cheeks, with impetigo behind the right ear, developed. The impetigo cleared with erythromycin, but the rash persisted despite topical steroids and took on an eczematoid appearance. Chest x-ray examination became negative 3 months after transplantation (Fig. 5).

MATERIALS AND METHODS

Serum and tear immunoglobulin levels were measured by single radial diffusion[10] using immunoglobulin standards certified by the World Health Organization. Immunoelectrophoresis was performed by the method of Scheidegger.[11] Tearing was induced with a salt crystal.[12] Genetic gamma-globulin typing for factors Gm(1), Gm(2), Gm(4) and Gm(5) and Inv(1) was done by inhibition of agglutination.[13]

The in vitro reactivity of lymphocytes to phytohemagglutinin was performed by addition of 0.01 ml of reconstituted PHA-M* to 0.1×10^6 of isolated peripheral lymphocytes and culture by the semimicroculture technic of Sengar and Terasaki.[14] After 72 hours, 0.5 μCi of tritiated thymidine was added, and the culture continued for 12 more hours. The DNA was then precipitated, solubilized and counted in a scintillation counter. Control cultures without phytohemagglutinin were run simultaneously. Normal lymphocytes activated with phytohemagglutinin incorporate 20 to 600 times more radioactive precursor than unstimulated lymphocytes.

*Difco Laboratories, Detroit, Mich.

16

Serotyping of peripheral lymphocytes of the patient and his family was performed by the microdroplet cytotoxicity test[15] with the use of a panel of 115 cytotoxic antiserums defining 25 specificities. Typing was performed on the patient's peripheral lymphocytes on 10 separate occasions before and eight occasions after transplantation, and thrice on bone-marrow aspirates after transplantation.

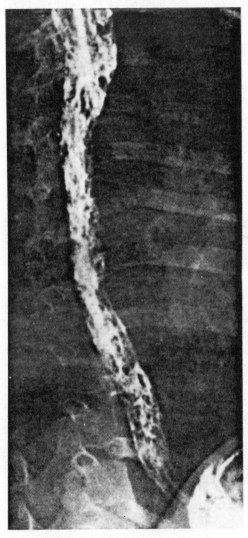

Figure 3. Barium Esophagram at 11 Months of Age, Revealing Mucosal and Submucosal Ulcerations of the Entire Esophagus, Compatible with the Clinical Diagnosis of Monilial Esophagitis.

On two occasions before transplantation mixed leukocyte cultures were performed by the semimicromethod of Sengar and Terasaki[14] on all the family members and unrelated persons.

Chromosome analyses of cultured peripheral lymphocytes, done by the method of Arakaki and Sparkes,[16] were performed on 10 separate occasions. Direct chromosome analysis on bone-marrow aspirates, done by the method of Tjio and Whang,[17] were performed on six separate occasions.

RESULTS

Immunoglobulins

The initial serum immunoglobulin levels at the age of five months disclosed an IgG of 100, IgM of 50 and IgA of less than 1 mg per 100 ml. Two weeks later, the IgG was 60, IgM 110, and IgA less than 1 mg per 100 ml. These levels are compatible with a diagnosis of severe antibody deficiency with some IgM synthesis intact. No tear immunoglobulins were detected on two occasions. Gamma-globulin injections or plasma infusions were given bi-

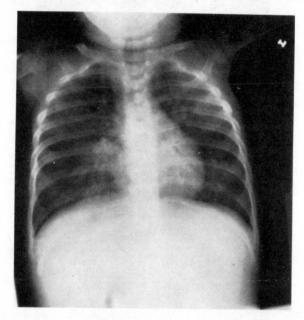

Figure 4. Chest Roentgenogram at the Age of 12 Months, One Month after Transplantation, at the Height of the Graft-versus-Host Reaction.

Since a needle aspirate and cultures were negative, a confluent infiltrate in the right middle or right lower lobe was attributed to a graft-versus-host response in the lung.

18

weekly during the next six months; the total immunoglobulin levels never exceeded 500 mg per 100 ml; most of this was attributable to exogenous gamma-globulin (Fig. 2).

Four weeks after transplantation, a sudden rise in all three immunoglobulins ensued, reaching a maximum total level of 2730 mg per 100 ml, eight weeks after transplantation. Immunoelectrophoresis of the patient's serum disclosed diffuse hypergammaglobulinemia rather than a single M-component. The immunoglobulins subsequently returned to normal levels for age.

During the GVH reaction, when marked conjunctivitis was present, tear immunoglobulins disclosed an IgG of 130, IgM of 71 and IgA of 20 mg per 100 ml. At this age the tear IgG level is normally 5 to 15, and the IgM less than 1 mg per 100 ml.[12] Two months later, after the GVH reaction and conjunctivitis had disappeared, the tear IgG was 15, tear IgM less than 1, and tear IgA 15 mg per 100 ml, which are normal values.

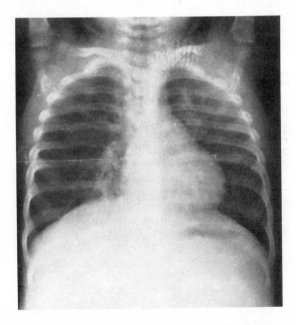

Figure 5. Chest Roentgenogram Two Months Later (at the Age of 14 Months).
The lung fields are clear except for minimal peribronchial changes remaining in the right lower lobe. There is still no thymic shadow.

19

Lymphocyte Studies

Phytohemagglutinin stimulation of the patient's lymphocytes on five occasions before transplantation showed no definite reaction as determined by thymidine incorporation into DNA. There was no response to mitomycin-treated allogeneic cells on two occasions before transplantation (Table 1). Five days after transplantation, the patient's lymphocytes were still nonreactive to PHA. Five weeks later, at the height of the GVH reaction, peripheral lymphocytes showed a moderate response to phytohemagglutinin (170 cpm resting and 4300 cpm stimulated). Thereafter, on five occasions during the period of clinical stabilization, reactivity increased to near normal values. On four occasions during the early post-transplantation period, unstimulated cultures of the patient's lymphocytes showed increased incorporation of thymidine above normal unstimulated lymphocytes.

HL-A Typing

Initial HL-A serotyping of the patient's lymphocytes disclosed several antigens (HL-A1, HL-A2, HL-A3, HL-A7, Te 40, Te 52, Te 54, Te 57, Te 59 and Te 63). Serotyping of the family indicated that the haptotype of the father was HL-A2, Te 54/HL-A3, HL-A7 and that of the mother HL-A2, Te 53/HL-A2, Te 55. Neither parent shared antigens HL-A1, Te 40, Te 59 or Te 63 with the patient. No blood transfusions had been administered to account for these antigens. None of the siblings had an HL-A type identical to the patient's. Repeat testing of the patient's lymphocytes on nine occasions before transplantation revealed 10 different antigens on one or more occasions.

At the age of 11 months, critical examination of the multiple results indicated that many of the antigenic specificities were found inconsistently and were not shared by either parent. This led to the conclusion that the patient genotypically had only three HL-A specificities (HL-A2, Te 52/HL-A2, Te 54) and that these were shared by the 12-year-old sister.

Mixed leukocyte cultures were then performed, and indicated that the patient's purified lymphocytes stimulated lymphocytes from all family members except from those of the 12-year-old sister, the eventual donor (Table 1).

After transplantation, extraneous antigens persisted although the donor's antigens (HL-A2, Te 52 and Te 54) were consistently present. During the GVH reaction, all the extraneous antigens disappeared, but they reappeared upon its subsistence. No antibodies to the extraneous antigens were ever detected. Bone-marrow HL-A typing after transplantation also showed multiple extraneous antigens. Attempts to type peripheral lymphocytes after culture with phytohemagglutinin were unsuccessful.

Chromosome Studies

Chromosome analysis of peripheral lymphocytes before transplantation could not be performed owing to lack of reactivity to phytohemagglutinin. This was also the situation five days after transplantation. However, chromosome analysis four weeks after transplantation and on five subsequent occasions disclosed an XX (donor) pattern.

The initial direct bone-marrow chromosome analysis performed five days after transplantation disclosed an XY pattern; one month later and on five subsequent occasions, all karyotypes were still XY.

Other Studies

Morphologic examination of the bone marrow disclosed the presence of well differentiated plasma cells beginning one month after transplantation. In one marrow aspirate, obtained five months after transplantation, there were a few clusters of lymphoblasts; these were not noted subsequently.

Genetic gamma-globulin typing of the patient's serum before gamma-globulin therapy was Gm(1)+, Gm(2)+,. Gm(4)−, Gm(5)− and Inv(1)−. After transplantation the typing was Gm(1)+, Gm(2)+, Gm(4)+, Gm(5)+ and Inv 1 (−) − a typing identical to that of the donor.

Poliomyelitis titers were negative before transplantation. Three months after transplantation, the titers were Type I, 1:128, Type II, 1:64, and Type III, 1:16. The donor's titers (she had received three oral poliomyelitis immunizations) were Type I, 1:16, Type II, 1:32, and Type III, 1:16.

Immediately after transplantation red-cell typing disclosed both donor (Rh-positive) and patient (Rh-negative) cells. The donor's cells diminished after that so that after two months, the majority (more than 95 per cent) of the erythrocytes were Rh negative.

DISCUSSION

Pretransplantation

The diagnosis of severe combined immunodeficiency was not immediately evident on initial presentation, despite the presence of thrush, primarily because of the patient's apparent well-being during the first months of life and at the time of examination, the equivocal family history of a similar disorder, the presence of small lymphocytes and the absence of lymphopenia. Lymphocyte counts averaged 4000 and never were less than 2500. Although lymphopenia is usually present in severe combined immunodeficiency, normal lymphocyte counts have been observed in several cases.[18]

The diagnosis was eventually established by low immunoglobulin levels, absence of antibody formation and failure of peripheral lymphocytes to respond to phytohemagglutinin. By that time, P. carinii pneumonia had been diagnosed by needle aspiration of the lung. This diagnosis must be suspected when pneumonia occurs in immunodeficiency since only pentamidine or pyrimethamine-sulfadiazine therapy is successful.[19,20] Our patient lived on a ranch and was exposed to numerous animals, natural reservoirs of P. carinii infection.[19]

Mycostatin was completely ineffective in controlling the oral moniliasis whereas gentian violet controlled but did not abolish it. The inability to control the moniliasis with leukocyte transfer factor from a monilia-sensitive donor or to convert any skin tests in our patient, unlike the successes reported in chronic mucocutaneous candidiasis[21] and the Wiskott-Aldrich syndrome,[22] indicates that the patient's small lymphocytes may be functionally impaired in terms of immunologic processing or mediator production, as in sarcoidosis.[23] When monilial esophagitis developed, intravenous amphotericin combined with continuous tube feeding was of benefit; however, amphotericin did not eradicate the oral moniliasis, indicating the special susceptibility of this location.

The extraneous HL-A types present on the patient's lymphocytes resulted in a delay in finding an HL-A identical donor. The sibling with identical mixed leukocyte culture and the patient had different HL-A typing on every occasion, a situation never previously encountered during our extensive experience correlating HL-A typing and mixed-leukocyte-culture results.[24,25] The simultaneous occurrence of more than four antigenic specificities on HL-A typing is also a most unusual finding and is at variance with current concepts of the HL-A antigens, which holds that each individual receives two genes from each parent controlling a maximum of four specificities. The only other two patients among 20,000 HL-A typings who had more than four specificities also had severe combined immunodeficiency.[26] This phenomenon has not been

22

noted in other patients with cellular or antibody-deficiency syndromes. These typing results may indicate the presence of antigenic determinants (possibly incomplete) on the cell surface, or a membrane abnormality characteristic of defective lymphocytes that renders them sensitive to certain typing serums and is unrelated to antigenic determinants on the cell. In favor of the latter interpretation is the fact that lymphocytes of the HL-A-identical sibling were not stimulated in mixed leukocyte culture by the patient's lymphocytes, despite antigenic disparity by lymphocyte typing, as discussed at greater length by Terasaki et al.[26]

When the patient's condition became critical and an HL-A identical donor was apparently unavailable, we decided to attempt a bone-marrow transplantation from a parent with concomitant use of antiserum to the patient's histocompatibility antigens as carried out by Buckley and her associates.[27] When repeat typing and mixed-leukocyte-culture tests identified the HL-A identical sibling, such an attempt was unnecessary. The clinical point from this experience is that in patients with severe combined immunodeficiency, if phenotypically excessive HL-A antigens are present, mixed leukocyte culture should be performed to aid in the identification of genotypically HL-A-identical siblings.

Transplantation

The marrow transplantation procedure was essentially that employed by the Minnesota group,[2,4,7] and consisted of the use of 2×10^9 unfractionated donor marrow cells given by the intraperitoneal route without concomitant transplantation of fetal thymus cells. In contrast to the advice of some authorities,[1] no attempt was made to isolate the patient, or to place him on prophylactic antibiotics during or immediately after transplantation; it seemed to us that the major infectious risks were from *P. carinii* organisms already present in his lung, *Candida albicans* already present in his mouth and gram-negative bacteria already present in his gastrointestinal tract. At the onset of the GVH reaction, when skin desquamation began, aseptic precautions as employed for burns were immediately instituted.

The severe GVH reaction that ensued was primarily manifested by cardiorespiratory symptoms, a finding prominent in only one[28] of the other bone-marrow transplantations with GVH reactions.[4,7,29] Because of the severity of the GVH reaction, we considered using methotrexate or antilymphocyte

23

serum, but these drugs were withheld because of the past failure in reversing an ongoing GVH reaction, the toxicity of these drugs in a sick and possibly septic infant, the poor prognosis if immunologic reconstitution was not achieved and the absence of reported fatalities in combined immunodeficiency from GVH attributable to an HL-A-identical marrow.

The transient disappearance of the extraneous HL-A types during the GVH reaction suggested elimination of host lymphocytes during this period. After subsidence of the reaction the extraneous antigens reappeared, suggesting that the patient's lymphocytes had returned to the circulation. This observation implies that the spontaneous cessation of the GVH reaction may have been associated with the acquisition of tolerance to the patient's tissues.

Post-transplantation

After cessation of the GVH reaction marked clinical improvement ensued at the same time as the occurrence of immunologic reconstitution. Evidence for engraftment was as follows: the increase in immunoglobulins and the appearance of isoagglutinins and poliomyelitis antibodies; the appearance of donor Gm type IgG-globulin in the patient's serum; the conversion of peripheral lymphocytes to a phytohemagglutinin-reactive state; the conversion of the monilia skin test to positive and disappearance of the moniliasis; and the presence of an XX (donor) pattern upon chromosomal analysis of peripheral lymphocytes.

The absence of XX (donor) cells upon direct (without phytohemagglutinin) analysis of the patient's bone marrow and the predominant Rh-negative (patient) red-cell type indicates that total replacement of the bone marrow with donor cells has not occurred. The presence of plasma cells in the bone marrow after transplantation, presumably of donor origin (because of the Gm-typing of the IgG-globulin) indicates partial engraftment. Plasma cells may represent a differentiated cell unable to proliferate and therefore unable to undergo mitosis for karyotyping. The precursor cells for the donor's lymphocyte in the circulation may be located in the liver, spleen, lymph nodes or lung.

The limited bone-marrow engraftment in this patient is similar to the findings now evident in the patient given a transplant by Bach and his associates over three years ago.[30] Their patient, a two-year-old boy, had immunodeficiency with thrombocytopenia and eczema (Wiskott–Aldrich syndrome),

615.36 Imbm
C.1

and transplantation of marrow from an HL-A-identical sister (whose karyotype was XXX) was successful. Eighteen days after the transplantation, one of six mitoses from the marrow disclosed XXX donor cells. Currently, no XXX cells are present in the marrow despite their continued presence in the peripheral blood and continued evidence of cellular immune reconstitution.[31] Three other patients with severe combined immunodeficiency who have received bone-marrow transplants also lack donor lymphocytes in the bone marrow (F. S. Rosen, personal communication), suggesting that this phenomenon is not uncommon.

We are indebted to Dr. Richard Hong, University of Wisconsin, for advice during many aspects of the patient's illness, to Dr. Marshall Goldberg, who referred the patient, to Dr. Phillip Sturgeon, who performed the Gm and red-cell typings, to Dr. Robert Sparkes and his associates of the Genetics Laboratory, who performed the chromosome studies, and to Drs. Eric Fonkalsrud and Richard Cahill, who assisted with the marrow transplantation.

REFERENCES

1. Fudenberg H, Good RA, Goodman HC, et al: Primary immunodeficiencies: report of a World Health Organization committee. Pediatrics 47:927-946, 1971
2. Gatti RA, Meuwissen HJ, Allen HD, et al: Immunological reconstitution of sex-linked lymphopenic immunological deficiency. Lancet 2:1366-1369, 1968
3. Buckley RH: Reconstitution: grafting of bone marrow and thymus: Progr Immunol (in press)
4. Meuwissen HJ, Gatti RA, Terasaki PI, et al: Treatment of lymphopenic hypogammaglobulinemia and bone-marrow aplasia by transplantation of allogeneic marrow: crucial role of histocompatibility matching. N Engl J Med 281:691-697, 1969
5. Gatti RA, Good RA: Follow-up of correction of severe dual system immunodeficiency with bone marrow transplantation. J Pediatr 79:475-479, 1971
6. De Koning J, Dooren LJ, Van Bekkum DW, et al: Transplantation of bone-marrow cells and fetal thymus in an infant with lymphopenic immunological deficiency. Lancet 1:1223-1227, 1969
7. Ammann AJ, Meuwissen HJ, Good RA, et al: Successful bone marrow transplantation in a patient with humoral and cellular immunity deficiency. Clin Exp Immunol 7:343-353, 1970
8. Bortin MM: A compendium of reported human bone marrow transplants. Transplantation 9:571-587, 1970
9. Rocklin RE, Chilgren RA, Hong R, et al: Transfer of cellular hypersensitivity in chronic mucocutaneous candidiasis monitored in vivo and in vitro. Cell Immunol 1:290-299, 1970
10. Stiehm ER, Fudenberg HH: Serum levels of immune globulins in health and disease: a survey. Pediatrics 37:715-727, 1966
11. Scheidegger JJ: Une micro-méthode de l'immuno-électrophorèse. Int Arch Allergy Appl Immunol 7:103-110, 1955
12. Stiehm ER, Miller A, Zeltzer PM, et al: Secretory defense system (SDS) in health and disease. Presented at the annual meeting of the Society for Pediatric Research, Atlantic City, New Jersey, April 28-May 1, 1971 .

25

13. Steinberg AG: Progress in the study of genetically determined human gamma-globulin types (the Gm and Inv groups). Progr Med Genet 2:1-33, 1962
14. Sengar DPS, Terasaki PI: A semimicro mixed leukocyte culture test. Transplantation 11:260-267, 1971
15. Mittal KK, Mickey MR, Singal DP, et al: Serotyping for homotransplantation. XVIII. Refinement of microdroplet lymphocyte cytotoxicity test. Transplantation 6:913-927, 1968
16. Arakaki DT, Sparkes RS: Microtechnique for culturing leukocytes from whole blood. Cytogenetics 2:57-60, 1963
17. Tjio JH, Whang J: Direct chromosome preparations of bone marrow cells, Human Chromosome Methodology. Edited by JJ Yunis. New York, Academic Press, 1965, pp 51-56
18. Hoyer JR, Cooper MD, Gabrielsen AE, et al: Lymphopenic forms of congenital immunologic deficiency diseases. Medicine (Baltimore) 47:201-226, 1968
19. Robbins JB: Pneumocystis carinii pneumonitis: a review. Pediatr Res 1:131-158, 1967
20. Kirby HB, Kenamore B, Guckian JC: Pneumocystis carinii pneumonia treated with pyrimethamine and sulfadiazine. Ann Intern Med 75:505-509, 1971
21. Schulkind ML, Adler WH, Altemeier WA, et al: Transfer factor in the treatment of chronic mucocutaneous candidiasis. Presented at the annual meeting of the Society for Pediatric Research, Atlantic City, New Jersey, April 28-May 1, 1971
22. Levin AS, Spitler LE, Stites DP, et al: Wiskott-Aldrich syndrome, a genetically determined cellular immunologic deficiency: clinical and laboratory responses to therapy with transfer factor. Proc Natl Acad Sci USA 67:821-828, 1970
23. Lawrence HS, Zweiman B: Transfer factor deficiency response — a mechanism of anergy in Boeck's sarcoid. Trans Assoc Am Physicians 81:240-248, 1968
24. Terasaki PI, Mickey MR: Histocompatibility-transplant correlation, reproducibility, and new matching methods. Transplant Proc 3:1057-1071, 1971
25. Bach FH, Day E, Bach ML, et al: Histocompatibility matching. V. A comparison of typing and mixed cultures in unrelated individuals. Tissue Antigens 1:39-46, 1971
26. Terasaki PI, Miyagima T, Sengar DPS, et al: Extraneous HL-A antigens in severe combined immunodeficiency disease. Transplantation (in press)
27. Buckley RH, Amos DB, Kremer WB, et al: Incompatible bone-marrow transplantation in lymphopenic immunologic deficiency: circumvention of fatal graft-versus-host disease by immunologic enhancement. N Engl J Med 285:1035-1042, 1971
28. Rubinstein A, Speck B, Jeannet M: Successful bone-marrow transplantation in a lymphopenic immunologic deficiency syndrome. N Engl J Med 285:1399-1402, 1971
29. Levey RH, Klemperer MR, Gelfand EW, et al: Bone-marrow transplantation in severe combined immunodeficiency syndrome. Lancet 2:571-575, 1971
30. Bach FH, Albertini RJ, Joo P, et al: Bone-marrow transplantation in a patient with the Wiskott-Aldrich syndrome. Lancet 2:1364-1366, 1968
31. Bach FH: Reconstitution by thymus, marrow, transfer factor and established lymphocytic cell lines, Immunologic Intervention. Edited by JW Uhr, M Landy. New York, Academic Press (in press)

26

FINE STRUCTURE OF THYMUS AFTER BONE MARROW TRANSPLANTATION IN AN INFANT WITH SEVERE COMBINED IMMUNODEFICIENCY

Dale E. Bockman, Ph.D., Alexander R. Lawton, M.D., and Max D. Cooper, M.D.

Patients with severe combined immunodeficiency (lymphopenic agammaglobulinemia or Swiss agammaglobulinemia) lack the capacity to express both cell-mediated (thymus-dependent) and humoral (thymus-independent) immune responses.[20] The developmental independence of these two systems has been demonstrated in animal models[10] and confirmed by analysis of certain congenital immune deficiency states in humans. Agenesis of the thymus and parathyroid glands (DiGeorge's syndrome) is characterized by severe impairment of cellular immune responses while immunoglobulin synthesis is normal. Restoration of the deficiency has been accomplished with fetal thymus transplants.[2, 8] Conversely, patients with the congenital sex-linked agammaglobulinemia of Bruton manifest normal cellular immune functions but lack the capacity to synthesize immunoglobulins (reviewed in Reference 9). On the basis of these observations, it has been postulated that the defect in patients lacking both limbs of immunity should be sought at the level of the lymphoid stem cell.[9] The fatal graft-*versus*-host disease which developed in earlier attempts to transplant bone marrow stem cells may be avoided by matching HL-A antigens.[3, 28] Recently, both cellular and humoral immune functions have been conferred on patients with lymphopenic agammaglobulinemia by transplantation of allogeneic bone marrow from HL-A identical siblings[1, 18, 32] or a stem cell-rich fraction of bone marrow and fetal thymus.[12] Thymus transplants alone have failed to induce immunocompetence in patients with lymphopenic agammaglobulinemia;[13, 21, 22, 24, 35, 36] the success obtained with hemopoietic cells thus support the hypothesis that the lymphoid stem cell is defective or absent in these patients.

The stem cell hypothesis implies that the thymus and the inductive site for differentiation of immunoglobulin-producing cells should be functionally intact in these patients. Thymic alymphocytosis, which has been the pathologic hallmark of this disease,[25] should be a secondary phenomenon, correctable by supplying an appropriate population of stem cells. The development of a mediastinal mass on x-ray 5 weeks after bone marrow transplantation in one infant provided circumstantial evidence that thymic lymphopoiesis had indeed been restored.[18]

The thymus of a patient with autosomal recessive lymphopenic agammaglobulinemia (Swiss agammaglobulinemia), in whom cellular and humoral immunity had been restored by bone marrow transplantation, is the focus of this report. The most striking finding was the paucity of lymphocytes in the thymus. This observation suggests that transfer of mature immunocompetent cells rather than differentiation of stem cells within the thymus accounted for development of cellular immune functions in this patient. The results of a comparison of the ultrastructural morphology of this patient with the fine structural features of 10 normal thymuses and a stress-involuted thymus are presented. Although the patient's thymus showed many fine structural alterations and initially led to skepticism concerning the functional integrity of the thymus in this disease, remarkably similar changes were found in the stress-involuted thymus. Restoration of thymic lymphopoiesis occurs rapidly after involution following irradiation or treatment with corticosteroids. Thus, the possibility exists that with a longer interval after bone marrow transplantation, thymic lymphoid population may be achieved.

MATERIALS AND METHODS

Subjects

Swiss Agammaglobulinemia Patient. A detailed report of the clinical and immunologic evaluation of this patient and the response to bone marrow transplantation is presented elsewhere.[30] Briefly, this white male infant developed oral and cutaneous candidiasis and rhinitis during the first weeks of life. Intermittent diarrhea began at 3 months of age. Agammaglobulinemia (immunoglobulin G (IgG) < 10 mg. per 100 ml., IgA and IgM undetectable) was diagnosed at 5 months following life-threatening pneumonia. The infant lacked isoagglutinins and did not respond to immunization with typhoid vaccine. Plasma

28

cells were not found by immunofluorescence or routine histologic techniques in biopsies of a lymph node and rectal mucosa. Lymphopenia (<2500 cells per cu. mm.) and total absence of circulating small lymphocytes were documented. A thymic shadow was not visualized. Few, if any, lymphocytes were present in the biopsied lymph node. Absence of functional cellular immunity was demonstrated by the failure of peripheral blood leukocytes to respond to phytohemagglutinin or allogeneic cells, delayed skin graft rejection (rejected only after bone marrow transplantation), absence of delayed cutaneous sensitivity to Candida antigen in the presence of Candida infection, and failure to develop a delayed reaction to keyhole limpet hemocyanin after immunization with this antigen. A female sibling of the patient had died at 6 weeks of age of overwhelming infection. Circulating lymphopenia and severe lymphoid depletion in lymph nodes and spleen examined at autopsy suggested that she and the propositus had the autosomal recessive type of lymphopenic agammaglobulinemia.

A 2-year-old immunologically normal brother served as the bone marrow donor. The donor and recipient were HL-A identical, except for a possible difference in the HL-A 4b antigen, but had different major blood group antigens. They were well matched by one-way mixed lymphocyte stimulation testing. Evidence of restoration of both cellular and humoral immune functions was obtained within 2 weeks of transplantation of 6.6 × 10^8 nucleated marrow cells. The skin graft was rejected, oral and cutaneous candidiasis cleared, the Candida skin test became positive, and normal numbers of lymphocytes, responsive to phytohemagglutinin stimulation, appeared in peripheral blood. Antibody synthesis was indicated by the appearance of a positive Coombs' test due to antibody with specificity for B cells (the patient was B, the donor A) and by rising serum levels of IgM. The patient survived a clinically mild graft-*versus*-host reaction but died of *Pneumocystis carinii* pneumonia 21 days after bone marrow transplantation. Peripheral lymphoid tissue obtained at autopsy contained many small lymphocytes, although fewer than normal. Follicular organization was lacking. Plasma cells were abundant in spleen, lymph nodes, and intestine. Cells containing IgM, IgG, and IgA were demonstrated by immunofluorescence.

Normal Human Thymus. Normal human thymus was taken from children and adults undergoing cardiac surgery. Small pieces of tissue were collected during preparation of the surgical field, fixed, and embedded for electron microscopic study as described below. The patients specifically used for illustrations in the present report include two children (5 years and 9 years old) and one adult (23 years old). A total of 10 subjects ranging in age from 5 through 57 years was available for comparison, however, and served as a base line for determining alterations.

Stress-Involuted Thymus. Involuted thymus came from a child who succumbed to overwhelming Gram-negative sepsis. This 11-month-old white male had bronchopneumonia accompanied by high fever in the range of 102–106° F. and rash over the face, trunk, and extremities for approximately 3 weeks prior to death. During this time there was a progressive decrease in the total white blood cell count and severe agranulocytosis developed. Pseudomonas, Aerobacter, and Klebsiella were cultured from the blood. Immunologic evaluation indicated a primary immune deficiency did not exist. Immunoglobulin levels were normal before death. Plasma cells containing IgM, IgG, and IgA were detected by immunofluorescent staining.

ELECTRON MICROSCOPY

Small fragments of thymus were fixed in Karnovsky's paraformaldehyde-glutaraldehyde fixative[27] buffered with *s*-collidine.[5] Tissue was maintained in collidine buffer for extended periods before postfixation in 2 per cent osmium tetroxide in phosphate buffer.[6] It was then left in 0.1 per cent aqueous uranyl acetate[29] overnight in the refrigerator before dehydration through graded ethanols and was embedded in Araldite[31] or Dow epoxy resin 334.[41] Sections were cut with a diamond knife on an LKB Ultratome III ultramicrotome. Thick (1 μ) sections were studied by light microscopy after staining with toluidine blue. Thin sections were mounted on uncoated copper grids, stained with lead citrate,[40] and examined with a Philips EM-300 electron microscope.

RESULTS

SWISS AGAMMAGLOBULINEMIA PATIENT

Location of thymic parenchyma for study was difficult because of the unusually high proportion of adipose connective tissue present in the tissue fragments. The amount of adipose connective tissue was more like that expected for an age-involuted thymus than in one from an infant. Moreover, normal architecture was not ob-

30

served when the islands of thymic parenchyma were studied by light microscopy (Fig. 1). There was a marked paucity of lymphoid cells. Epithelial cell nuclei and smaller, dense nuclei of uncertain identity were present in high proportion. Scattered accumulations of histiocytes with mixed, dense staining and light, circular granules were prominent.

Electron microscopic examination of the histiocytes (Fig. 2) revealed in many a dense population of heterogeneous lipochrome pigment granules. Large, roughly circular profiles of electron-lucent material within the histiocytes had the appearance of individual droplets of neutral lipid. This appearance is identical with that of cells

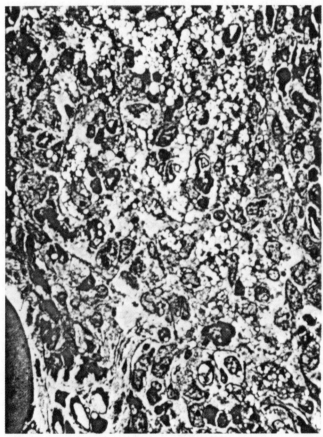

Fig. 1. Thymus from patient with Swiss-type agammaglobulinemia 21 days after bone marrow transplant. Part of a fat cell appears at *lower left*. Note paucity of lymphoid cells and abundance of histiocytes with multiple clear, circular inclusions. Epoxy section stained with toluidine blue; ×800.

31

recently described in the lymph node of a patient with familial lipochrome histiocytosis by Clawson, Rodey, and Good[7] except that we did not observe Langerhans granules in the present study.

Only scattered lymphoid cells were observed by electron microscopy (Fig. 2). Some of these had the ultrastructural appearance of typical small lymphocytes. Others (inset, Fig. 2), although having lymphoid characteristics, had more cytoplasmic granules, filaments, and lipid inclusions than is usual for small lymphocytes. In this respect, they resembled the cells observed in the patient's peripheral blood before bone marrow transplantation.[30] Larger lymphoid cells or blast cells were not observed.

The epithelial framework (Figs. 3–5) was also atypical. The relative lack of lymphocytes caused an apparent packing together of epithelial cells in islands separated from the abundant surrounding connective tissue by a continuous basal lamina (Figs. 3 and 4). The epithelial cell-connective tissue boundary was very irregular. Epithelial cells typically had a relatively small, dense nucleus surrounded by a moderate amount of dense cytoplasm. Particularly dense bundles of tonofilaments were abundant in the cytoplasm (Figs. 3–5). Desmosomes occurred at epithelial junctions.

Two types of extracellular substance were observed within the epithelial islands. One type obviously represented continuations of the connective tissue extending inward between epithelial cells (Figs. 3–5). The other type, a moderately dense, flocculent material (Figs. 3 and 5), had a less obvious origin. The presence of fibrils within the flocculent material, the reduplication of basal lamina within some extensions of connective tissue space, and the continuity of basal lamina and flocculent material (Fig. 5) led to the conclusion that the second type of extracellular substance represented extension of connective tissue space to which had been added considerable quantities of excess basal lamina material.

No Hassall's corpuscles were observed. Yet the lobular architecture, the position in the mediastinum, and the ultrastructural appearance of epithelial cells, as compared with the appearance of lymph nodes in other areas, clearly identified this as thymic tissue despite its highly abnormal structure.

NORMAL HUMAN THYMUS

Location of thymic parenchyma in normal children (Figs. 6–8) presents no problem since there is little adipose tissue within the gland. Lymphocytes in varying stages of maturation are quite numerous (Figs. 6 and 7). A variety of epithelial cells, joined with each other by desmosomes, is evident. Three varieties of epithelial cell from the thymus of a 5-year-old child are illustrated in Figures 6 and 7. The central epithelial cell in Figure 6, with a large oval nucleus containing delicate, evenly distributed chromatin and an electron-lucid cytoplasm, is a type not uncommon in normal thymus. The same may be said for the large, darker epithelial cell shown in Figure 7. Neither of these cell types was observed, however, in either the Swiss agammaglobulinemia patient or the patient with stress-involuted thymus.

The border of epithelial cells with connective tissue is characteristically very regular in normal thymus (Figs. 6 and 8). A single, regular basal lamina parallels epithelial cell membrane at this border.

Tonofilaments were evident in epithelial cell cytoplasm (Fig. 8). They are prominent in the areas of desmosomes. Small bundles of tonofilaments were present in some areas of the cytoplasm of epithelial cells, but never to the extent observed in the Swiss agammaglobulinemia patient. The exception to this was the large bundles of tonofilaments always present in epithelial cells of Hassall's corpuscles (Fig. 9). These dense bundles seemed comparable to those in thymic epithelial cells of the immune deficient patient, even though no Hassall's corpuscles were present in that patient.

STRESS-INVOLUTED THYMUS

Thymic morphology in this individual was strikingly similar to that observed in the Swiss agammaglobulinemia patient. Adipose connective tissue was prominent. Islands of thymic parenchyma contained few lymphocytes. There were more lymphocytes, however, than in the Swiss agammaglobulinemia patient.

Hassall's corpuscles with characteristic morphology were present. Epithelial cells unassociated with Hassall's corpuscles showed increased concentrations of tonofilaments. The varied morphology typical of epithelial cells in normal thymus was not observed; this was similar to the narrowed range of epithelial cell morphology in the Swiss agammaglobulinemia patient. The border between epithelial cells and connective tissue was very irregular (Figs. 10 and 11). The associated basal lamina followed this irregularity (Fig. 10) and frequently was reduplicated and extremely tortuous (Fig. 11). Extensions of connective tissue space between thymic parenchyma showed the same irregularities of basal lamina and expansion of

33

basal lamina material (Fig. 12) as has been described for the Swiss agammaglobulinemia patient.

Numerous lipid-laden histiocytes (Fig. 13), identical in fine structure with those in the Swiss agammaglobulinemia patient, were present.

DISCUSSION

By light microscopy, the morphologic features of the thymus from the child with severe combined immunodeficiency were identical with those described previously in patients with this entity not given bone marrow transplants.[25] At the electron microscopic level, this thymus was markedly different from the normal thymus in the present study and from normal human fetal and infant thymus as described by others.[19, 23, 26, 34] The high proportion of adipose tissue as compared with thymic parenchyma is more characteristic of an aged, involuted thymus. Lymphocytes normally should comprise a considerable proportion of thymic parenchyma; their paucity was striking and in some cases their cytologic features were atypical. Further, many of the lymphocytes were located in the connective tissue space outside the basal lamina rather than within the thymic epithelial cell reticulum.

The epithelial cells which provide the framework within which lymphopoiesis normally occurs were much more dense and compact than usual. The prominent bundles of tonofilaments in their cytoplasm are more typical of epithelial cells at the periphery of Hassall's corpuscles than those in association with developing lymphocytes. Yet Hassall's corpuscles were not observed in the Swiss agammaglobulinemia patient. It is impossible to determine from the present study alone whether numerous lymphocytes were present in the interstices between epithelial cells and subsequently were removed or whether epithelial cells did not develop normally because lymphoid cells were not differentiating within their framework.

Two observations from the present investigation should be kept in mind for comparison with future studies on thymic abnormalities associated with the autosomal recessive form of severe combined immunodeficiency and other immune deficiency states: the unusually large concentrations of basal lamina material and the macrophages which were so prominent in certain areas.

Pierce and Nakane[33] convincingly demonstrated marked changes in epithelial basement membranes in response to injury produced by x-irradiation, chemicals, and bacteria. X-ray-induced glomerulosclerosis in mice, for instance, was found to be the result of accumulation of basement membrane (basal lamina) material between the mesangial cells. Ross and Grant,[37] studying changes in rat testicular tissue after hypophysectomy, showed duplication, folding, and distortion of the basal lamina in response to atrophy of the epithelium with which it was associated. In our Figure 5 is shown a combination of folding, reduplication, and excessive accumulation of basal lamina material in the Swiss agammaglobulinemia patient. This is consistent with, but does not prove, the possibility that the thymus in this patient was at one time larger than at the time of study. The presence of lymphoid cells in epithelial cell interstices would make the thymus larger. The involuted thymus in the present study, which presumably had normal morphology at one time, appeared almost identical so far as basal lamina abnormalities were concerned.

The fine structure of the lipid-laden macrophages observed in the present study appears quite similar to that described for histiocytes in the spleen of a patient with fatal granulomatous disease of childhood[4] and in the lymph node of a patient with familial lipochrome histiocytosis.[7] Unfortunately, the precise nature of the basic defect in these diseases is not known, so little inference can be drawn to explain the appearance of such cells in the present study. The similarity should be noted, however, and remain as part of the data which hopefully will lead to an understanding of the specific disease states and the general reactions which they represent.

The thymus is highly sensitive to steroid hormone levels.[14] Experimental involution of thymus by hydrocortisone[11] or testosterone[16] leads to a relative depletion of lymphoid cells and considerable phagocytosis of degenerating cells. Debris-laden histiocytes are thus a common element in rapidly involuting thymus, as might be produced by stress. Thymic involution produced by endotoxin produces these cells.[17] The vacuolated large phagocytic cells shown by Frey-Wettstein and Craddock[16] in an Epon-embedded $1\text{-}\mu$ section of testosterone-treated rat thymus are quite similar to the histiocytes observed in the present study. Smith[38] has characterized cells in mouse thymus which are ultrastructurally identical with the lipid-laden macrophages described in this report, and has called them lipopigment cells.

Partial restoration of thymus-dependent immune responses occurred following bone marrow transplantation in the patient with combined immunodeficiency. Nevertheless, significant lymphoid population of the thymus

35

was not found at postmortem examination 3 weeks after the marrow graft. Ford et al.[15] have observed a similar delay in seeding of grafted bone marrow cells to the thymus of lethally irradiated mice; a plateau in numbers of donor cells was reached only after about 3 months. These observations suggest that restoration of thymus-dependent immune responses resulted from the adoptive transfer of immunocompetent lymphocytes rather than differentiation of stem cells within the thymus. Whether longer exposure to stem cells would result in thymic lymphopoiesis must be determined after long term study of other patients.

Another explanation of the fine structural observations on the thymus from the patient with severe combined immunodeficiency cannot be ruled out by the present study. Although distinguished morphologically by a larger lymphocyte population and the presence of Hassall's corpuscles, the stress-involuted thymus in this study was strikingly similar to the thymus from the patient with combined immunodeficiency in regard to reduplication of the basal lamina, the prominence of lipopigment cells, and the narrowed spectrum of epithelial cell morphology. It is not impossible that the thymus was populated by stem cells and that some differentiation took place before subsequent involution was caused by the stress of the transient graft-versus-host disease and fatal Pneumocystis carinii pneumonia. Proving or disproving this possibility would necessitate biopsies before, and at intervals after, transplantation. Nevertheless, this possibility seems unlikely since both population and subsequent involution of the thymus in the patient would have to have taken place within 21 days. Conversely, Ford et al.[15] showed a marked delay in seeding of bone marrow cell to the thymus as compared with other tissues of experimental animals.

Although we found no morphologic evidence that the thymus had received stem cells of donor bone marrow origin and influenced them to begin lymphoid development in situ, humoral factors produced by the patient's thymus could have enhanced development and function of donor postthymic cells elsewhere in the body.[39] It will be of interest to examine "thymus hormone" production in these patients, when assays become available for man, particularly since normal production would provide additional support for the idea that the potential for normal thymus function exists in severe combined immunodeficiency. Apart from the absence of Hassall's corpuscles, structures that follow lymphoid population even in nor-

36

mal thymus development, our morphologic studies failed to reveal any abnormalities of the epithelial thymus proper that could not be due entirely to stress. While such stress effects on the thymus probably would have at least temporary deleterious effects on its function, our observations appear to be consistent with the idea that, given time, the thymus in a patient with severe combined immunodeficiency could receive bone marrow stem cells and foster their normal development along immunocompetent lymphoid lines.

Acknowledgments. Normal human thymus was obtained through the cooperation of W. Arnold McAlpine, M.D., Hugh M. Foster, M.D., and Morris W. Selman, M.D.

This investigation was supported by Grants AM13535, AI08345, and M01RR3210 from the United States Public Health Service and by the American Cancer Society.

REFERENCES

1. Ammann, A. J., Meuwissen, H. J., Good, R. A., and Hong, R. Successful bone marrow transplantation in a patient with thymic hypoplasia and combined system immunologic deficiency. *Clin. Exp. Immunol. 7:* 343, 1970.
2. August, C. S., Rosen, F. S., Filler, R. M., Janeway, C. A., Markowski, B., and Kay, H. E. M. Implantation of a foetal thymus, restoring immunological competence in a patient with thymic aplasia (DiGeorge's syndrome). *Lancet 2:* 1210, 1968.
3. Bach, F. H., Albertini, R. J., Joo, P., Anderson, J. L., and Bortin, M. M. Bone-marrow transplantation in a patient with the Wiskott-Aldrich syndrome. *Lancet 2:* 1364, 1968.
4. Bartman, J., Van de Velde, R. L., and Friedman, F. Pigmented lipid histiocytosis and susceptibility to infection: ultrastructure of splenic histiocytes. *Pediatrics 40:* 1000, 1967.
5. Bennett, H. S., and Luft, J. H. *s*-Collidine as a basis for buffering fixatives. *J. Biophys. Biochem. Cytol. 6:* 113, 1959.
6. Clark, S. L., Jr. The thymus in mice of strain 129/J, studied with the electron microscope. *Am. J. Anat. 112:* 1, 1963.
7. Clawson, C. C., Rodey, G. E., and Good, R. A. Ultrastructure of familial lipochrome histiocytosis. *Lab. Invest. 22:* 294, 1970.
8. Cleveland, W. W., Fogel, B. J., Brown, W. T., and Kay, H. E. M. Foetal thymic transplant in a case of DiGeorge's syndrome. *Lancet 2:* 1211, 1968.
9. Cooper, M. D., Gabrielsen, A. E., and Good, R. A. Role of the thymus and other central lymphoid tissues in immunological disease. *Ann. Rev. Med. 18:* 113, 1967.

37

10. Cooper, M. D., Perey, D. Y., Peterson, R. D. A., Gabrielsen, A. E., and Good, R. A. The two-compartment concept of the lymphoid system. In *Immunologic Deficiency Diseases in Man*, edited by Bergsma, D. New York, The National Foundation, 1968.
11. Cowan, W. K., and Sorenson, G. D. Electron microscopic observations of acute thymic involution produced by hydrocortisone. *Lab. Invest. 13:* 353, 1964.
12. deKonig, J., Dooren, L. J., van Bekkum, D. W., van Rood, J. J., Dicke, K. A., and Radl, J. Transplantation of bone-marrow cells and fetal thymus in an infant with lymphopenic immunological deficiency. *Lancet 1:* 1223, 1969.
13. Dooren, L. J., deVries, M. J., van Bekkum, D. W., Cleton, F. J., and deKonig, J. Sex-linked thymic epithelial hypoplasia in two siblings. Attempt at treatment by transplantation with fetal thymus and adult bone marrow. *J. Pediatr. 72:* 51, 1968.
14. Dougherty, T. F. Effect of hormones on lymphatic tissue. *Physiol. Rev. 32:* 379, 1952.
15. Ford, C. E., Micklem, H. S., Evans, E. P., Gray, J. G., and Ogden, D. A. The inflow of bone marrow cells to the thymus: studies with part-body irradiated mice injected with chromosome-marked bone marrow and subjected to antigenic stimulation. *Ann. N. Y. Acad. Sci. 129:* 283, 1966.
16. Frey-Wettstein, M., and Craddock, C. G. Testosterone-induced depletion of thymus and marrow lymphocytes as related to lymphopoiesis and hematopoiesis. *Blood 35:* 257, 1970.
17. Gad, P., and Clark, S. L., Jr. Involution and regeneration of the thymus in mice, induced by bacterial endotoxin and studied by quantitative histology and electron microscopy. *Am. J. Anat. 122:* 573, 1968.
18. Gatti, R. A., Meuwissen, H. J., Allen, H. D., Hong, R., and Good, R. A. Immunological reconstitution of sex-linked lymphopenic immunological deficiency. *Lancet 2:* 1366, 1968.
19. Goldstein, G., Abbot, A., and Mackay, I. R. An electron-microscope study of the human thymus: normal appearances and findings in myasthenia gravis and systemic lupus erythematosus. *J. Pathol. Bacteriol. 95:* 211, 1968.
20. Good, R. A., Peterson, R. D. A., Perey, D. Y., Finstad, J., and Cooper, M. D. The immunological deficiency diseases of man: consideration of some questions asked by these patients with an attempt at classification. In *Immunologic Deficiency Diseases in Man*, edited by Bergsma, D. New York, The National Foundation, 1968.
21. Greenberg, A. H., Ray, M., and Tsai, Y. T. Thymic alymphoplasia and dysgammaglobulinemia type I. *J. Pediatr. 75:* 97, 1969.
22. Harboe, M., Pande, H., Brandtzaeg, P., Tveter, K. J., and Hjort, P. F. Synthesis of donor type γG-globulin following thymus transplantation in hypo-γ-globulinemia with severe lymphocytopenia. *Scand. J. Haematol. 3:* 351, 1966.
23. Hirokawa, K. Electron microscopic observation of the human thymus of the fetus and the newborn. *Acta Pathol. Jap. 19:* 1, 1969.
24. Hitzig, W. H., Kay, H. E. M., and Cottier, H. Familial lymphopenia with agammaglobulinaemia: an attempt at treatment by implantation of foetal thymus. *Lancet 2:* 151, 1965.
25. Hoyer, J. R., Cooper, M. D., Gabrielsen, A. E., and Good, R. A. Lymphopenic forms of congenital immunologic deficiency diseases. *Medicine (Baltimore) 47:* 201, 1968.

26. Kameya, T., and Watanabe, Y. Electron microscopic observations on human thymus and thymoma. *Acta Pathol. Jap. 15:* 223, 1965.
27. Karnovsky, M. J. A formaldehyde-glutaraldehyde fixative of high osmolality for use in electron microscopy. *J. Cell Biol. 27:* 137A, 1965.
28. Kay, H. E. M. Concepts of cellular deficiency and replacement therapy in immune deficiency. In *Immunologic Deficiency Diseases in Man*, edited by Bergsma, D., p. 168. New York, The National Foundation, 1968.
29. Kellenberger, E., Ryter, A., and Séchaud, J. Electron microscope study of DNA-containing plasms. II. Vegetative and mature phage DNA as compared with normal bacterial nucleoids in different physiological states. *J. Biophys. Biochem. Cytol. 4:* 671, 1958.
30. Lawton, A. R., III, Bockman, D. E., and Cooper, M. D. Treatment of autosomal recessive lymphopenic agammaglobulinemia by transplantation of matched allogeneic bone marrow. *Am. J. Med.*, in press.
31. Luft, J. H. Improvements in epoxy resin embedding methods. *J. Biophys. Biochem. Cytol. 9:* 409, 1961.
32. Meuwissen, H. J., Gatti, M. D., Terasaki, P. I., Hong, R., and Good, R. A. Treatment of lymphopenic hypogammaglobulinemia and bone-marrow aplasia by transplantation of allogeneic marrow. *N. Engl. J. Med. 281:* 691, 1969.
33. Pierce, G. B., and Nakane, P. K. Basement membranes. Synthesis and deposition in response to cellular injury. *Lab. Invest. 21:* 27, 1969.
34. Pinkel, D. Ultrastructure of human fetal thymus. *Am. J. Dis. Child. 115:* 222, 1968.
35. Rosen, F. S., Gitlin, D., and Janeway, C. A. Alymphocytosis, agammaglobulinemia, homografts, and delayed hypersensitivity: study of a case. *Lancet 2:* 380, 1962.
36. Rosen, F. S., Gotoff, S. P., Craig, J. M., Ritchie, J., and Janeway, C. A. Further observations on the Swiss type of agammaglobulinemia (alymphocytosis). The effect of syngeneic bone marrow cells. *N. Eng. J. Med. 274:* 18, 1966.
37. Ross, M. H., and Grant, L. On the structural integrity of basement membrane. *Exp. Cell Res. 50:* 277, 1968.
38. Smith, C. Studies on the thymus of the mammal. XVI. Lipopigment cells in the cortex of the thymus of the mouse. *Am. J. Anat. 124:* 389, 1969.
39. Stutman, O., Yunis, E. J., and Good, R. A. Studies on thymus function. II. Cooperative effect of newborn and embryonic hemopoietic liver cells with thymus function. *J. Exp. Med. 132:* 601, 1970.
40. Venable, J. H., and Coggeshall, R. A simplified lead citrate stain for use in electron microscopy. *J. Cell Biol. 25:* 407, 1965.
41. Winborn, W. B. Dow epoxy resin with triallyl cyanurate, and similarly modified Araldite and Maraglas mixtures, as embedding media for electron microscopy. *Stain Technol. 40:* 227, 1965.

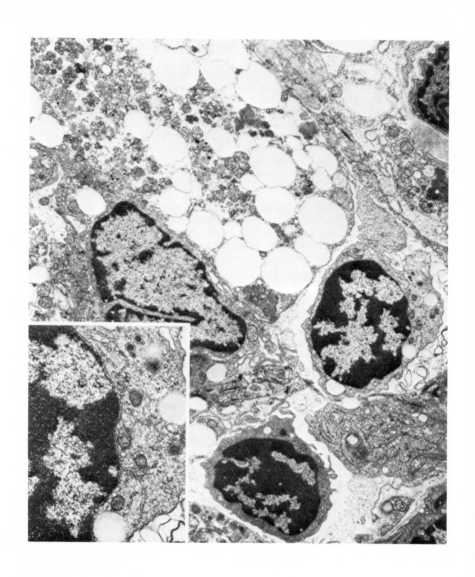

Fig. 2. Electron micrograph of a histiocyte within thymic parenchyma of Swiss agammaglobulinemia patient. Heterogeneous granules and larger, lighter lipid droplets are packed in the cytoplasm.
Two lymphoid cells adjoin the histiocyte. *Inset*, Higher magnification of one of the lymphoid cells, showing granules, filaments, and
lipid droplets in the cytoplasm. Figure 2, ×10,000; *inset*, ×26,000.

41

FIG. 3. Swiss agammaglobulinemia patient. Thymic epithelial cells at junction with connective tissue. A basal lamina, in some places reduplicated (*arrow*), occurs along the border. Extensions of connective tissue (*E*) and extracellular flocculent material (*O*) are evident. Capillary at *lower left.* ×11,000.

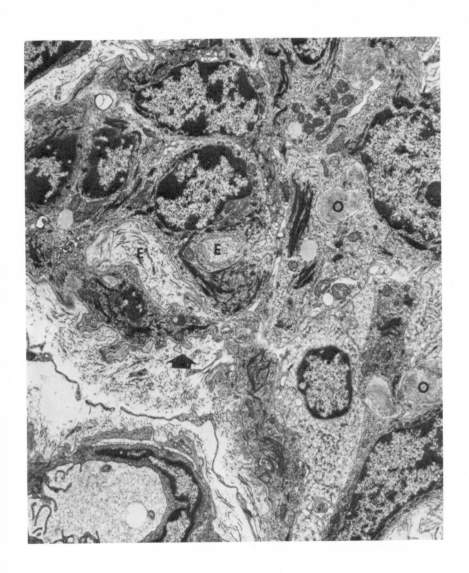

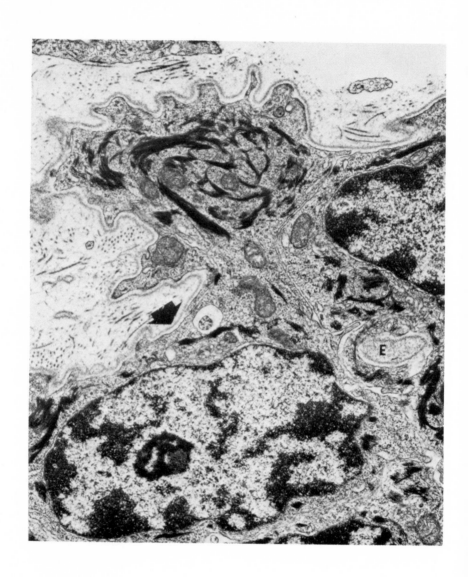

FIG. 4. Swiss agammaglobulinemia. Higher magnification of epithelial cell-connective tissue interface. Basal lamina (*arrow*) is shown to better advantage than in previous figure. An inward extension of connective tissue (*E*) and dense bundles of tonofilaments are evident. ×25,000.

FIG. 5. Swiss agammaglobulinemia. Extension of connective tissue at *upper left* shows reduplication of basal lamina (*solid arrow*). *Open arrow* indicates junction of basal lamina and flocculent material (*O*). Cytoplasmic clumps of tonofilaments are distributed about the central epithelial nucleus. ×16,000.

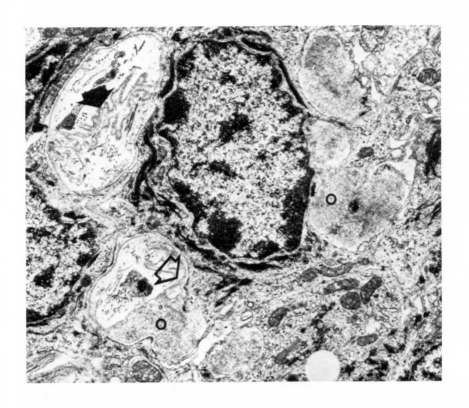

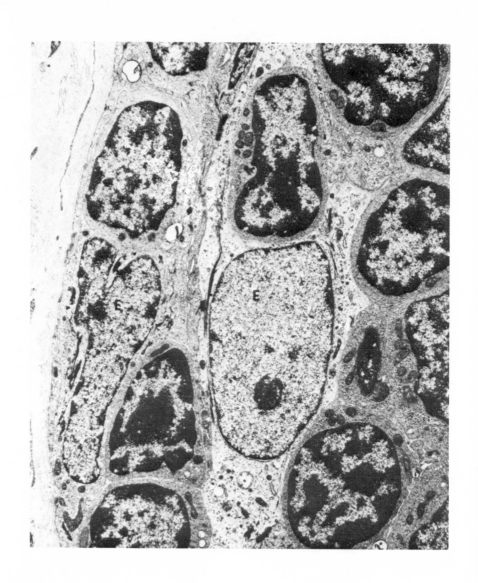

FIG. 6. Thymus from normal 5-year-old. Numerous lymphocytes are present. Two epithelial cell nuclei (E) are shown. Note that the epithelial cell on the *left* and attenuated extensions from adjacent epithelial cells form a regular border in contact with connective tissue. The basal lamina is smooth and single. The central epithelial cell has a large, open nucleus, prominent nucleolus, and light cytoplasm with few tonofilaments. ×11,000.

Fig. 7. Thymus from same individual as Figure 6. An epithelial cell (*E*) with scanty cytoplasm is surrounded by lymphocytes. The epithelial cell nucleus is large, elongate, and angular. Small patches of chromatin are dispersed through the nuclear profile. ×9,000.

Fig. 8. Junction of epithelial cell with connective tissue in thymus of normal 9-year-old. Note the large nucleus with dispersed chromatin and prominent nucleolus. A few thin tonofilaments are present. The cell border and basal lamina are regular. Capillary at *upper left*. ×19,000.

Fig. 9. Portion of Hassall's corpuscle from normal 23-year-old. The bundles of tonofilaments are comparable to those common in epithelial cells of Swiss agammaglobulinemia patient (compare with Figure 4). ×19,000.

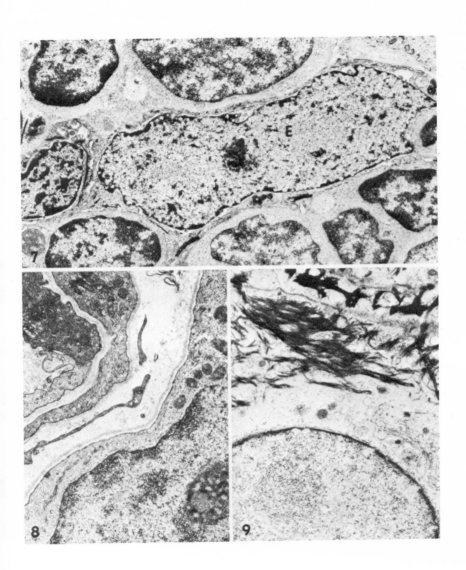

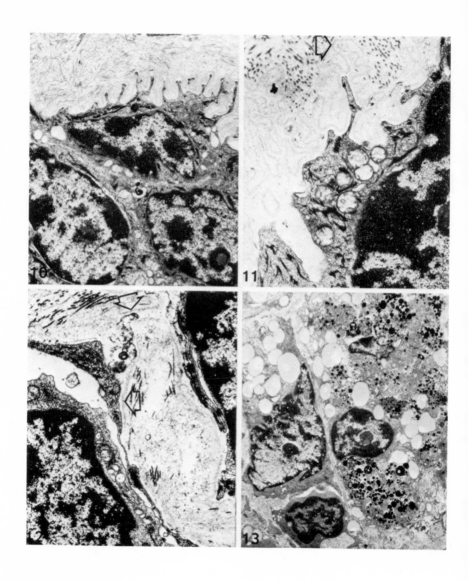

FIG. 10. Epithelial cells at their junction with connective tissue in patient with stress-involuted thymus. Nuclear chromatin and cytoplasm are condensed. Bundles of tonofilaments are evident. Cell border and basal lamina are irregular. ×11,000.

FIG. 11. Same patient as Figure 10. Epithelial cell-connective tissue interface. Basal lamina (*arrow*) is tortuous and reduplicated. ×22,000.

FIG. 12. Stress-involuted thymus. Basal lamina material (*arrows*) is continuous with gray, flocculent material occupying an extension of connective tissue space. Compare with Figure 5. ×19,000.

FIG. 13. Stress-involuted thymus. Lipid-laden macrophages (histiocytes and lipopigment cells) identical with those from Swiss agammaglobulinemia patient (**Figure 2**). ×6,000.

Review of Bone Marrow Transplants at the Ontario Cancer Institute

D. Amato, D. E. Bergsagel, A. M. Clarysse, D. H. Cowan,
N. N. Iscove, E. A. McCulloch, R. G. Miller, R. A. Phillips,
A. H. Ragab and J. S. Senn

Bone marrow transplantation cannot be widely applied for the treatment of various human diseases until the risk of graft-versus-host disease (GVHD) is minimized. Since the pluripotent stem cells required for permanent engraftment and the lymphoid cells responsible for GVHD have different physical properties, cell separation offers an attractive method for obtaining populations of stem cells free from cells that cause GVHD. The group at Rijswijk has used density separation to obtain populations enriched with stem cells.[1] They have used this enriched fraction to restore immunological function in a child with Swiss-type agammaglobulinemia.[2]

Our experience with various types of cell separation indicated that separation on the basis of cell size might be a more efficient method than density for separating stem cells from lymphoid cells. Separations on the basis of size are easily achieved by the method of velocity sedimentation.[3] Experiments with mouse bone marrow showed that it was possible by this method to recover a fraction with 70 per cent of the stem cells and only 5 per cent of the cells

Supported by Ontario Cancer Treatment and Research Foundation Grant 159.

that cause GVHD.[4] Cells from this stem cell-rich fraction were transplanted into lethally irradiated, allogeneic recipients and no signs of acute GVHD were observed. Interested members of the Department of Medicine and the Division of Biological Research of the Ontario Cancer Institute agreed to collaborate in the application of these findings to man.

Tests with human bone marrow showed that the cells capable of forming colonies in culture (CFU-C) could be separated by velocity sedimentation from the cells that reacted to phytohemagglutinin (PHA) or in mixed leukocyte culture.[5] If the former measurement can be used as an assay for stem cells and the latter for immunologically competent cells, these results indicate that velocity sedimentation gives the desired separation of stem cells from the immunologically competent cells in human bone marrow.

On the basis of these results it was decided to proceed with a clinical test of the separation procedure. The first requirement in setting up the clinical experiment was to develop a system capable of processing the large number of cells required for transplantation. After collection of the bone marrow and aspiration of buffy coats, one usually has approximately 3×10^{10} total cells, of which approximately one third are nucleated cells. To process this number of cells, two large sedimentation vessels (40 cm. in diameter) were constructed (Corning Glassware of Canada, Ltd.). Each chamber has a capacity of 18 liters and can be used to process a maximum of 1.3×10^{10} total cells. For separation the cells are suspended in 2500 ml. of Ringers saline with 0.3 per cent human serum albumin (HSA), and introduced into the bottom of the sedimentation vessel. A gradient of 1 to 2 per cent HSA in Ringers is then in-

55

troduced slowly into the chamber. As the gradient is formed, the cells are gradually raised to the top of the chamber, where they form a band 2 cm. thick. The cells are allowed to sediment in the cold for 12 hours at which time there is a clear separation into two bands, a rapidly sedimenting band containing mostly granulocytes and CFU-C and a slowly sedimenting band containing erythrocytes, nucleated erythrocytes and lymphocytes. Fractions of 200 ml. are then collected and the cells counted with an electronic cell counter. The cell counter is also attached to a pulse-height analyzer for the determination of the distribution of cell volumes in each fraction. The decision concerning the fractions to pool for transplantation is made on the basis of the volume distributions. All of the fractions containing predominantly large cells are pooled for transplantation. Tests using fresh cadaver bone marrow showed that the large chambers gave separations with resolution comparable to that obtained with the smaller chambers.[6]

This method of cell separation has been tested in three patients—two adults with acute leukemia and one child with Swiss-type agammaglobulinemia. The results are summarized in Table 1. The first patient, a 26-year-old woman with acute myeloblastic leukemia, received a transplant when she failed to respond to conventional chemotherapy. She was pretreated with donor blood followed by cyclophosphamide as described by Santos et al.[7] and then given the stem cell fraction of bone marrow from an HL-A identical brother. She died of a ruptured mycotic aneurism in her splenic artery 17 days after transplantation. At the time of death there was no evidence of GVHD nor was there any indication that the transplanted bone marrow was functioning; only XX karyotypes were found in

Table 1.—Summary of Bone Marrow Transplants at the Ontario Cancer Institute

Patient	Disease	Treatment	Donor	Number of Cells Transplanted	Take	GVH	Status
27 years—♀	Acute myeloblastic leukemia	Cyclophosphamide	Brother—HL-A identical	2.5×10^9	?	No	Died 17 days; ruptured mycotic aneurism
32 years—♂	Acute lymphoblastic leukemia	Cyclophosphamide	Brother—HL-A identical	2.5×10^9	Yes	Mild	Died 77 days; pneumonia
2 months—♂	Swiss-type agamma-globulinemia	None	Mother	1.4×10^9	No	No	Died 52 days; respiratory insufficiency

a bone marrow aspirate taken 2 days before death. At autopsy large numbers of leukemic cells were found in the femur, indicating that the cyclophosphamide probably did not kill all the leukemic cells.

The second patient to receive fractionated bone marrow was a 32-year-old man with acute lymphoblastic leukemia. At the time of transplantation he was in remission that had been induced with L-asparaginase. He was pretreated with cyclophosphamide as before and also received the stem cell fraction from an HL-A identical brother. Following transplantation there was a brief period of marked leukopenia during which the patient had a high fever and was treated with antibiotics. Thirteen days after transplantation his peripheral white blood cell count began to increase, and at the same time he developed a generalized erythematous rash. As his peripheral white blood cell count increased, his fever improved. By the 26th day after transplantation his temperature had returned to normal, and antibiotic therapy was discontinued. However, throughout this period, his rash continued and on the 23rd day became desquamative. At the same time he had a short episode of diarrhoea. Although these symptoms may be indicative of a mild GVHD, a skin biopsy was not typical of GVHD. His liver function tests have shown only slight deviation from normal throughout the posttransplant period. On the 28th day he developed a pronounced eosinophilia, which persisted for 17 days. Peripheral blood leukocytes first became responsive to phytohemagglutinin in culture 20 days after transplantation. At 35 days, donor erythrocytes were detected in the peripheral blood. The donor was Fy[a] positive and the recipient negative; density separation on the 35th day showed that the lightest, i.e., the youngest,[8] red blood cells were the ones that contained the Fy^a antigen. On the basis of these data, we make the tentative conclusion that transplantation of separated bone marrow cells has led to a successful bone marrow graft with only minimal GVHD.

The third patient[5] was a two-month-old male infant with Swiss-type agammaglobulinemia in Winnipeg, Manitoba. This child did not have a suitable HL-A identical donor, and bone marrow was taken from his mother. Because of the child's condition at the time of transplantation, the mother came to Toronto, the marrow was processed and the pooled stem cell fraction was flown to Winnipeg where it was transfused into the recipient. Transportation of the cells to Winnipeg caused only a 5-hour delay in the time which the cells were given as compared with our previous transplants, but a dye exclusion test immediately before transplantation showed that 95 per cent of the cells in the pool excluded trypan blue, indicating little loss in viability. Previous tests on this infant indicated that no immunosuppressive therapy was needed. Two weeks after birth he received a skin graft from an unrelated donor; at the time of the bone marrow transplant the skin graft had not been rejected. Although the child has remained free of infections since transplantation, there has been no evidence of a take in this patient: only male karyotypes are present in the bone marrow; the skin graft from the unrelated donor is intact; skin tests are negative, and immunoglobulin levels have not increased. There has also been no evidence of GVHD.

Although more testing is required, this method of cell separation appears to offer a simple and reproducible method for obtaining large numbers of stem cells for transplantation. The absence of GVHD in the child with Swiss-type agammaglobulinemia who received HL-A incompatible bone marrow from his mother, indicates the efficiency with which lymphoid cells can be removed from suspensions of bone marrow by this method of cell separation.

ACKNOWLEDGMENTS

The HL-A typing was done by Dr. S. Sekiguchi of Toronto Western Hospital. Tests for the Fy^a antigen were made by Mrs. Marie Crookston of Toronto General Hospital. The transplant on the 2-month-old infant with Swiss-type agammaglobulinemia was carried out in collaboration with Dr. John Foerster in Winnipeg.

REFERENCES

1. Dicke, K. A., van Hooft, J. I. M., and van Bekkum, D. W. Transplantation 6:571, 1968.

2. de Koning, J., Dooren, L. J., van Bekkum, D. W., van Rood, J. J., Dicke, K. A., and Radl, J. Lancet 1:1223, 1969.

3. Miller, R. G., and Phillips, R. A.: J. Cell. Physiol. 73:191, 1969.

4. Phillips, R. A., and Miller, R. G.: J. Immun. (in press).

5. Amato, D., Iscove, N. N., Cowan, D. H., and McCulloch, E. A.: Exp. Hemat. 20:8, 1970.

6. Amato, D., Cowan, D. H., and Phillips, R. A.: Proc. Can. Fed. Biol. Soc. 13:130. 1970.

7. Santos, G. W., Sensenbrenner, L. L., Burke, P. J., Colvin, O. M., Owens, A. H., Jr., Bias, W., and Slavin, R.: Exp. Hemat. 20:78, 1970.

8. Lief, R. C., and Vinograd, J.: Proc. Nat. Acad. Sci. USA 51:520, 1964.

SUCCESSFUL BONE MARROW TRANSPLANTATION IN A PATIENT WITH HUMORAL AND CELLULAR IMMUNITY DEFICIENCY

A. J. AMMANN, H. J. MEUWISSEN, R. A. GOOD
AND R. HONG*

SUMMARY

An immunity deficiency disease occurring in three siblings is described. Two siblings, a boy and a girl, died at ages $1\frac{1}{2}$ years and $4\frac{1}{2}$ years respectively with overwhelming varicella, varicella pneumonia and sepsis. Their disease included thymic hypoplasia, lymphopenia, deficient humoral and cellular immunity, absent serum IgA, neutropenia and eosinophilia.

Transplantation of bone marrow, identical by cytotoxic and mixed leucocyte assay, red cell antigens and Gm and Inv factors was given to an affected girl from a normal sibling on two occasions. The first transplant given at 6 months of age resulted in clinical improvement of the patient and some evidence of immunologic reconstitution. Complete correction of the immunity defect was achieved following a second bone marrow transplant at 11 months of age. A delayed onset and prolonged course of GVH reaction was observed following the second transplant. The patient survived the GVH without specific therapy. Evidence for complete immunologic reconstitution continued to be present 1 year following the second transplantation.

INTRODUCTION

Transplantation of allogeneic bone marrow to immunity deficient subjects has rarely been accomplished. To date, evidence for reconstitution has been presented in two cases of lymphopenic hypogammaglobulinaemia (Gatti et al., 1968; de Konig et al., 1969), and a patient with Wiskott-Aldrich syndrome (Bach et al., 1968). We report successful bone marrow transplantation in a girl with an autosomal form of thymic hypoplasia associated with lymphopenia, neutropenia, eosinophilia, absent cellular immunity and deficient antibody formation. Two siblings, a male age $1\frac{1}{2}$ years and a female age $4\frac{1}{2}$ years, died from overwhelming varicella infection and sepsis and were shown to have IgA deficiency (Hoyer et al., 1967).

* R.H. is a career development awardee of the USPHS.

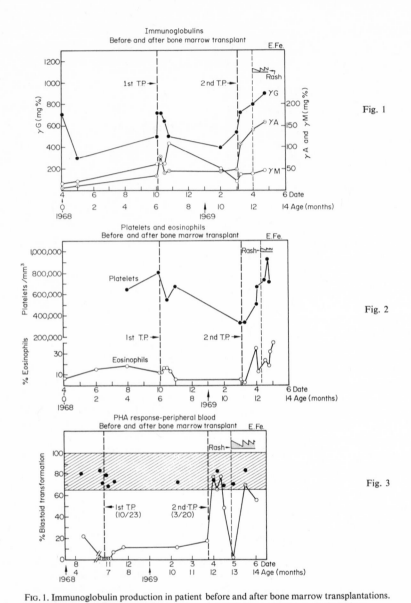

FIG. 1. Immunoglobulin production in patient before and after bone marrow transplantations.
FIG. 2. Platelet and eosinophil counts before and after bone marrow transplantations.
FIG. 3. PHA response of peripheral lymphocytes before and after bone marrow transplantations.

Case Report

E.F., a female infant, was first evaluated at 2 weeks of age. The only positive physical finding was a mild seborrheic rash. Laboratory studies revealed a haemoglobin of 18 g/100 ml, white blood cell count (WBC) 6850/mm³ with 33% polymorphonuclears, 49%

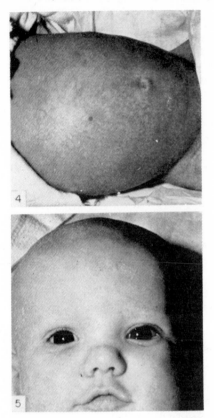

Fig. 4. Rash on patient at 6 months of age. Note maculopapular appearance and fine desquamation.

Fig. 5. Patient at 6 months of age. Note absence of hair and eyebrows.

lymphocytes, 11% monocytes and 7% eosinophils. Immunoglobulins were (mg/100 ml), IgG 700, IgM < 2, IgA < 2 (Fig. 1). The lymphocytes responded subnormally to phytohaemagglutinin (PHA). Subsequently, the lymphocytes became completely unresponsive to PHA (Fig. 3). Peripheral eosinophilia and thrombocytosis appeared (Fig. 2). No thymus shadow was seen on tomograms of the mediastinum. Over the next 6 months a maculopapular erythematous, desquamating eruption appeared, initially involving only the scalp and then spreading to the entire body (Fig. 4). Hair on the scalp and eyebrows became scant (Fig. 5).

At 6 months of age the patient was admitted to the University of Minnesota Hospitals for detailed immunologic evaluation and possible bone marrow transplantation. The physical examination revealed a chronically ill infant. She was in the 10th percentile for height and weight. The skin was as previously described.

Studies (summarized in Table 1) showed deficient humoral and cellular immunity. A bone marrow biopsy revealed megakaryocytosis, eosinophilia and the presence of plasma cells. Biopsy of a stimulated node showed generalized depletion of lymphocytes and poor follicular formation (Fig. 6). Rectal biopsy showed increased numbers of plasma cells and inflammatory cells. The skin showed slight lymphoid infiltration of the epidermis and vacuolization in the basal cell layer.

TABLE 1. Immunologic function before and following first and second bone marrow transplantation

Time	Age (months)	Small lymphs (%)	PHA	DNFB†	Isohaemagglutinins titre
Before transplant	6	2	0*	negative	0
After 1st transplant	7–11	5	15	positive	0
After 2nd transplant	12	14	100	positive	1:4

* Per cent transformation. † Positive skin response to challenge dose following sensitization.

A normal 6-year-old sister (the only surviving sibling) was found to be histocompatible with the patient as determined by cytotoxic assay and mixed leucocyte culture.

The patient received an intraperitoneal infusion of 45 ml of bone marrow from the normal sibling consisting of approximately 1.25×10^3 nucleated cells. The marrow was collected as described previously (Gatti et al., 1968).

Over the next 5 months the patient improved. Some evidence of engraftment was provided by the following observations: 1—increased responsiveness of the lymphocytes to PHA stimulation although this response still did not reach normal intensity (Fig. 3), 2—development of cutaneous reactivity to DNFB (Table 1), 3—the amelioration of the skin rash (see below). A decrease in the peripheral eosinophilia (Fig. 2) and generalized improvement in the appetite and disposition occurred. Nevertheless, no specific humoral antibody responses could be demonstrated (Table 1). These findings were interpreted as an indication that only partial immunologic reconstitution had been accomplished. Accordingly a second bone marrow transplantation from the same donor was performed at 11 months of age. Marrow from the normal HL-A matched sibling was again utilized. At this time 153 ml of bone marrow containing approximately 9×10^9 nucleated cells were given. In order to minimize dilution of the bone marrow by peripheral blood no more than 3 ml was taken from any one site. No adverse reactions were observed in the donor or host as a consequence of the transplant. One week following the second transplant the eosinophils decreased to 2%, the platelets decreased to 326,000, the lymphocytes now transformed normally when stimulated by PHA, and the immunoglobulins were (mg/100 ml) IgG720 IgM 43, IgA 110

(Figs. 1, 2, 3). Evidence for further immunologic reconstitution following this marrow transplant was thus obtained.

The patient continued to do well until the 40th day following the second transplant.

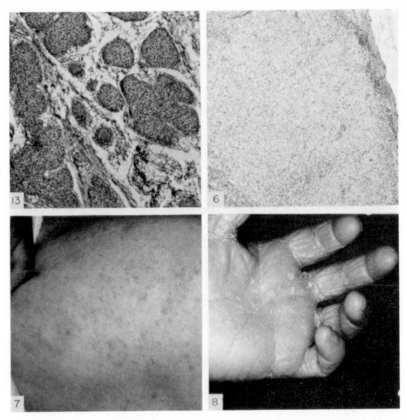

FIG. 13. Thymus (× 32 magnification, H and E stain) of Je.F., brother of the patient, showing absence of corticomedullary differentiation and Hassel's corpuscles.

FIG. 6. Stimulated lymph node (× 32 magnification, H and E stain), showing generalized lymphoid depletion and lack of follicle formation.

FIG. 7. Generalized maculopapular rash 40 days following second transplant.

FIG. 8. Hand of patient 8 weeks following second transplant showing waxy appearance and desquamation.

At this time a faint erythematous, maculopapular rash was observed primarily on the trunk. During the following weeks the rash increased in severity and extent (Fig. 7) and was associated with eosinophilia and thrombocytosis (Fig. 2). It was felt at this time that the patient was experiencing a mild graft versus host (GVH) reaction. Over the next 4 weeks an episode of otitis media, upper respiratory illness, and DPT immunization, each occurring as separate events, resulted in an exacerbation of the rash, eosinophilia and thrombocytosis. Eight weeks foliowing the second transplant the patient was admitted to the hospital with fever and cough. Physical examination revealed erythematous, waxy skin with marked

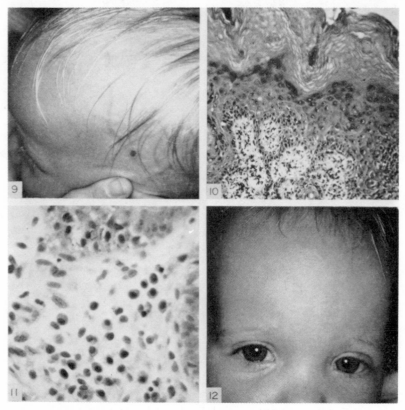

FIG. 9. Patient 8 weeks following second transplant showing loss of hair.

FIG. 10. Skin biopsy (× 80 magnification, H and E stain) taken during GVH showing lymphocyte infiltration, basal cell vacuolization, dyskeratosis and epidermal thickening.

FIG. 11. Rectal biopsy (× 340 magnification, H and E stain) during GVH showing increased plasma cells and inflammatory cells.

FIG. 12. Patient 12 weeks following second transplant showing growth of scalp hair, eyebrows and eyelashes.

desquamation (Fig. 8), loss of hair (Fig. 9), eyebrows, and eyelashes and splenomegaly. Laboratory studies revealed a 40% eosinophilia, 926,000 platelets/ml^3, increased orinithine carbamyl transferase (OCT) of 40 deca units, white cells which reduced nitroblue tetrazolium (NBT) and a normal electrocardiogram. Perihilar infiltrate was present in the chest

X-ray. A lung biopsy demonstrated increased number of alveolar macrophages and a mononuclear cell infiltrate. Silver and Giemsa stains did not reveal Pneumocystis carinii organisms. A skin biopsy revealed marked epidermal infiltration with lymphocytes, basal cell layer vacuolization, dyskeratosis and epidermal thickening, all characteristic of a graft versus host reaction (Fig. 10).

Thirteen weeks following the second transplant the patient continued to show desquamation of the skin and had several febrile episodes with temperatures up to 104–105°F. Prednisone (5 mg/day) was given in an attempt to decrease the GVH reaction. However, because of hypertension (160/110), the steroid was discontinued after 3 days. Nevertheless, gradual improvement occurred with a cessation of desquamation of the skin, no further hair loss, return of temperature to normal and decrease of platelets, eosinophil counts and OCT to normal. Hypertension persisted to a mild degree but the etiology remained obscure despite extensive studies. Urinalyses were always normal and renal function tests, intravenous pyelogram, urinary catecholamines and metanephrines were all normal. The patient did not exhibit any gastrointestinal tract symptoms during the entire GVH reaction. A rectal biopsy showed increased numbers of inflammatory and plasma cells (Fig. 11). The only indication of liver involvement was the transitory elevation of the OCT.

Gradual improvement in the patient continued. Twelve weeks following the second transplant no evidence of skin rash was present and scalp hair, eyebrows, eyelashes and new nail growth was present (Fig. 12). Diffuse skin pigmentation was observed. Hypertension gradually decreased and was normal 20 weeks following the second transplant. The patient continues to do well 1 year following the second transplant.

Siblings of patient

Je.F., the sister of the patient, was evaluated at age $2\frac{1}{2}$ years for recurrent otitis media. Initial studies revealed lymphopenia, neutropenia and eosinophilia. Between the ages of 2 and 4 years she had numerous episodes of fever, otitis media and pneumonia. Death occurred at $4\frac{1}{2}$ years following severe varicella complicated by varicella, pneumonia and staphylococcal sepsis. Absence of serum IgA was demonstrated at this time.

An autopsy showed a small thymus with absence of Hassall's corpuscles, lymphoid depletion, and absence of corticomedullary differentiation (Fig. 13). The lymph nodes showed marked depletion of lymphocytes in the thymic dependent area (paracortical). Plasma cells were abundant and normal primary and secondary follicular formation was seen. Ischemic necrosis with type-A intranuclear inclusions were observed throughout the viscera.

Ed.F., the brother of the patient, contracted varicella at the same time as his sister and died from an overwhelming infection with varicella pneumonia and pseudomonas sepsis. The patient was shown to have lymphopenia, neutropenia, eosinophilia and absent serum IgA. An autopsy revealed essentially similar findings to Je.F. In addition, inclusions characteristic of cytomegalic inclusion cell disease were observed. These two patients were reported in detail in a previous communication (Hoyer *et al.*, 1967).

DISCUSSION

Immunologic reconstitution of our patient was achieved utilizing two separate allogeneic bone marrow transplants from a normal sibling shown to be identical to the patient at the

HL-A locus by cytotoxic assay (Terasaki, Vredevoe & Mickey, 1967), and mixed leucocyte culture (Bach & Voynow, 1966). In addition the patient and sibling were determined to be identical in the major and minor blood groups and Gm and Inv factors tested.

A bone marrow transplant of $1 \cdot 25 \times 10^9$ nucleated cells was given at 6 months of age. Immunologic reconstitution was inadequate following the first transplant but some signs of improvement were noted: 1—improved disposition and appetite, 2—gradual fading and disappearance of rash, 3—appearance of scalp hair, eyebrows and eyelashes, 4—return to normal of platelets and eosinophils, 5—response to PHA, although suboptimal, 6—positive skin reaction to DNFB. Our interpretation of these events is that in the first transplant of immunocompetent cells and stem cells too few cells were given. In addition, the marrow was obtained from only two sites and most likely was diluted with peripheral blood.

After the second graft was given (5 months following the first transplant, age 11 months) evidence for further immunologic reconstitution was obtained. The lymphocytes transformed normally when stimulated by PHA, isohaemagglutinins were present (Table 1) and the immunoglobulins increased to (mg/100 ml) IgG 720, IgM 43, IgA 110 (Fig. 1). As the patient and the donor were identical in all antigens tested and both were females, no markers were present to permit detection of donor cells. The disposition and appearance of the patient continued to improve and weight gain was observed.

Spontaneous improvement is a consideration but we know of no cases of spontaneous conversion of a cellular immunity defect. Further, it seems unlikely that all of the tests of immunologic function could have reverted to normal in a period of 1 week as a matter of coincidence. The persistence of these responses and the continued increase of immunoglobulin levels indicates that this was not simply a passive transfer of immunocompetent cells but a true engraftment and establishment of a replicating cell line. In addition, the presence of a prolonged GVH reaction indicated persistence of the immunity defect of the host cells.

Because most GVH reactions occur 1–2 weeks following transplantation (Hathaway et al., 1966; Rosen et al., 1966; Miller, 1967), it was felt that our patient had passed the critical period. However, 40 days following the second transplant the first evidence of GVH appeared.

The diagnosis of GVH mediated by immunocompetent donor cells was based on the characteristic skin rash (Fig. 7) and skin biopsy showing lymphocyte infiltration of the epidermis, dyskeratosis, basal cell vacuolization and thickening of the epidermis (Fig. 10), (Kodawaki et al., 1965). In addition, loss of hair, eyebrows, eyelashes, fever, thrombocytosis, eosinophilia and elevated liver enzymes occurred. Although more severe than observed in our previous case, the GVH was not fatal and spontaneously improved without significant therapy. It seems to us unlikely that the brief period of prednisone therapy had a significant influence on the course. During the entire course of the GVH a positive NBT test ($>25\%$ reduction) was observed. This test which depends on the reduction of NBT by cells which are actively phagocytizing is usually negative in viral infections ($<10\%$ reduction) but positive in bacterial infections (Park, Fikrig & Smith, 1968; Park et al., 1969). It is unlikely that active bacterial infection could have been present in the patient for a period of 3 months (all cultures were normal and a lung biopsy for Pneumocystis carinii was negative). Since NBT reduction is also seen in the phagocytosis of particulate matter (Windhorst et al., 1968), it is possible that the destruction of host cells occurring during a GVH reaction yields products which are eliminated by a phagocytic mechanism and could account for the positive NBT test. The exacerbation of the GVH reaction on three separate occasions by either infection (upper respiratory infection, otitis media) or DPT antigen is of great interest. One can only speculate as to the mechanism involved, however it is possible that in all three instances antigenic stimulation of immunocompetent cells could have produced factors which exacerbated the GVH reaction non-specifically, e.g. by means of macrophage proliferation with production of factors involved in inflammatory reactions (Keller, 1968; Schild & Willoughby, 1967).

In addition to the delayed onset of the GVH (40 days) in our patient, a prolonged course was observed. The prolonged course may have been due to the large number of immunocompetent cells given in the second transplant. The delayed onset and prolonged course may also be related in some as yet unknown way.

Modification of the GVH has been attempted by several different means. Theoretically the transplant should contain only the desired stem cells. Separation of stem cells from other immunocompetent cells which could participate in the GVH reaction has been attempted utilizing an albumin gradient (de Konig et al., 1969). Nevertheless the patient described in whom successful marrow transplantation was achieved with such a preparation also experienced a mild GVH reaction. Pretreatment with immunosuppressive agents has been advocated, based upon experience in animal experimentation (Thomas et al., 1962), but limited use of these agents in man has not yet proved effective (Mathe et al., 1969). Antilymphocyte serum treatment of the donor marrow was utilized in one of our previous cases but experience with this method in man is also limited. Careful antigenic matching is a necessity if GVH reaction is to be avoided or kept to a minimum in bone marrow transplantation. In our patient identity of the recipient with the donor was established utilizing a cytotoxic assay (Terasaki et al., 1967), and mixed leucoyte culture (Bach & Voynow, 1966). Not all white cell antigens are detected by these techniques however, and further, the sensitivity of the mixed leucocyte culture is insufficient to indicate differences in minor (non HL-A) loci. Currently a 'mild' GVH reaction may have to be accepted as an unavoidable complication of bone marrow transplantation prior to the establishment of a tolerant state. We believe that optimal testing includes evidence of donor and host match on both cytotoxic and mixed leucocyte assays. Of the two assay systems the mixed leucocyte culture seems more discriminating since antigenic differences may be detected by this method which cannot yet be detected by cytotoxic assay.

Severe GVH reactions are associated with characteristic features such as skin rash, fever, hepatosplenomegaly, diarrhoea and jaundice. In our patient skin rash was the predominant feature. No gastrointestinal tract symptomatology nor jaundice was present and fever, splenomegaly and elevated liver enzymes were only transiently present. Hair loss, not previously emphasized in man but a predominant feature in protracted GVH in animals appeared to be an important feature of the GVH reaction in our case. Return of hair and nail growth coincided with improvement in the patient. In addition, certain laboratory studies appear to be sensitive indicators of the onset and severity of the GVH. Eosinophilia and thrombocytosis preceded clinical symptomatology of GVH, increased with the severity of the GVH, and returned to normal more slowly than the clinical findings. It is possible that thrombocytosis may be an early and sensitive indicator of GVH. The finding of thrombocytosis in autoimmune disease (Bean, 1965) indicates that intense immunologic reactivity may be associated with this phenomenon.

The long term effects and complications of chronic GVH are unknown. Although our patient is currently doing well, low grade hypertension persisted for several months perhaps representing a complication of GVH reactions in those who survive. Renal involvement in fatal GVH has been described (Miller, 1967); however, our patient had normal renal function tests and urinalysis. A renal biopsy was not performed.

Certain features of the patient's initial presentation suggest that a GVH reaction may have been present shortly after birth. The diffuse maculopapular rash was similar to that observed following the second transplant which resulted in a GVH reaction. The patient also lacked scalp hair, eyebrows and eyelashes. A rectal biopsy showed inflamatory cell infiltrate in the mucosa and blood eosinophilia and thrombocytosis were present. Following the first transplant, hair, eyebrow and eyelash growth occurred and the skin rash resolved. Eosinophilia and thrombocytosis decreased (Fig. 2). The initial findings were interpreted as evidence of a GVH reaction, the graft being of maternal origin. The clinical picture was highly reminiscent of the case reported by Kodawaki et al. (1965). Also consistent with a GVH reaction in early life was the finding of low levels of all three immunoglobulins rather than the pattern of IgA deficiency seen in the two other siblings. In Kodawaki's case, it was suggested that the graft was able to produce small amounts of immunoglobulins. Unfortunately, no erythrocyte or γ-globulin antigenic markers could be employed in our case to verify this assumption.

The exact classification of the immunologic defect in the patient and her siblings is difficult. The syndrome consists of thymic hypoplasia, isolated IgA deficiency, lymphopenia, neutropenia, eosinophilia and defective humoral and cellular immunity. It is not apparent what form of inheritance exists in these patients but the involvement of both male and female siblings in a single generation would be compatible with autosomal recessive inheritance.

The ethical and legal implications of bone marrow donation from children is a subject of proper concern. Several aspects of marrow transplantation make its utilization different from that of organ transplantation. So far as is currently known, the removal of bone marrow has no detrimental effect on the donor, and further, unlike removal of organs, leaves the donor with a remaining replicating cell population. Although the use of non-sibling donors has resulted in some successful renal transplants (Barnes, 1965), bone marrow transplantations from non-siblings have resulted either in failure of engraftment or fatal GVH reactions.

ACKNOWLEDGMENT

This work was aided by National Foundation, USPHS-A1-08677, HE-06314 and A1-07726.

REFERENCES

BACH, F.H., ANDERSON, J.L., ALBERTINI, R.J., JOO, P. & BORTIN, M.M. (1968) Bone marrow transplantation in a patient with the Wiskott–Aldrich syndrome. Lancet, ii, 1364.
BACH, F.H. & VOYNOW, N.K. (1966) One-way stimulation in mixed leukocyte cultures. Science, 153, 545.
BARNES, B.A. (1965) Survival data of renal transplantations in patients. New Engl. J. Med. 272, 776.
BEAN, R.H.O. (1965) Thrombocytosis in auto-immune disease. Bibl. haemat. (Basel), 23, 43.
DE KONIG, J., DOOREN, L.J., VAN BEKKUM, D.W., DICKE, K.A., VAN ROOD, J.J. & RADL, J. (1969) Transplantation of bone marrow cells and fetal thymus in an infant with lymphopenic immunological deficiency. Lancet, i, 1223.
GATTI, R.A., MEUWISSEN, H.J., ALLEN, H.D., HONG, R. & GOOD, R.A. (1968) Immunological reconstitution of sex-linked lymphopenic immunological deficiency. Lancet, ii, 1366.

HATHAWAY,W.E., BRANGLE, R.W., NELSON, T.L. & ROECKEL,J.E. (1966)Aplastic anemia and alymphocytosis in an infant with hypogammaglobulinemia: Graft-versus-host reaction? *J. Pediat.* **68,** 713.

HOYER, J.R., COOPER, M.D., GABRIELSEN, A.E. & GOOD, R.A. (1967) *Immunologic Deficiency Diseases in Man* (Ed. by D. Bergsma and R. A. Good), pp. 91–103. New York. Birth Defects: Original Articles Series.

KELLER, R. (1968) On the role of secondary mast-cell damage and histamine-release in the course of immune reactions. In CIOMS Int. Sym. Biochem. *Acute Allergic Reactions,* pp. 253–264. Blackwell Scientific Publications, Oxford.

KODAWAKI, J., ZUELSER, W.W., BROUGH, A.J., THOMPSON, R.I., WOOLEY, P.V. & GRUBER, D. (1965) XX/XY lymphoid chimerism in congenital immunological deficiency syndrome with thymic alymphoplasia. *Lancet,* ii, 1152.

MATHE, G., AMIEL, J.L., SCHWARTZENBERG, L., SCHNEIDER, M., CATTAN, A., SCHLUMBERGER, J.R., NOUZA, K. & HRASK, K. (1969) Bone marrow transplantation in man. *Trans. Proc.* **1,** 16.

MILLER, M.E. (1967) Thymic dysplasia ('Swiss agammaglobulinemia'). I. Graft-versus-host reaction following bone marrow transfusion. *J. Pediat.* **70,** 730.

PARK, B.H., FIKRIG, S.M. & SMITHWICK, E.M. (1968) Infection and nitrobluetetrazolium reduction by neutrophils. *Lancet,* ii, 532.

PARK, B.H., HOLMS, B.M., RODEY, G.E. & GOOD, R.A. (1969) Nitroblue-tetrazolium test in children with fatal granulomatous disease and newborn infants. *Lancet,* i, 157.

ROSEN, F.S., GOTOFF, S.P., CRAIG, J.M., RITCHIE, J. & JANEWAY, C.A. (1966) Further observations on the Swiss type of agammaglobulinemia (alymphocytosis). The effect of syngeneic bone marrow cells. *New Engl. J. Med.* **274,** 18.

SCHILD, H.O. & WILLOUGHBY, D.A. (1967) Possible pharmacological mediators of delayed hypersensitivity. *Brit. med. Bull.* **23,** 46.

TERASAKI, P.I., VREDEVOE, D.L. & MICKEY, M.R. (1967) Serotyping for homotransplantation. X. Survival of 196 grafted kidneys subsequent to typing transplantation. *Transplantation,* **5,** 1057.

THOMAS, E.D., COLLINS, J.A., HERMAN, E.C. & FERREBEE, J.W. (1962) Marrow transplants in lethally irradiated dogs given methotrexate. *Blood,* **19,** 217.

WINDHORST, D.B., PAGE, A.R., HOLMS, B., QUIE, P.G. & GOOD, R.A. (1968) The pattern of genetic transmission of the leukocyte defect in fatal granulomatous disease of childhood. *J. clin. Invest.* **47,** 1026.

Application of Marrow Grafts in Human Disease

George W. Santos, MD

THE INITIAL DISCOVERY of Jacobson *et al* [1] in 1949 that mice could be protected from an otherwise lethal dose of x-ray by lead shielding of the spleen led to the subsequent observation of others that a variety of lethally x-irradiated mammals could be saved from death by intravenously injecting syngeneic, allogeneic or in some cases xenogeneic marrow suspensions. [2] These initial observations provided the laboratory worker with the stimulus and much of the methodology for further fundamental investigations into the areas concerned with the differentiation and kinetics of hematopoietic stem cells, kinetics of antibody formation, thymus-marrow interactions, etc. The clinician was no less excited by these early observations because of the obvious implications of therapy for human disease. The majority of early attempts at marrow grafting in man failed, [3] however, because of lack of knowledge regarding tissue typing, immunosuppression and experience in the supportive care of patients with bone marrow aplasia. With new knowledge in these areas, there has been a resurgence of interest in the application of marrow grafts in human disease. [4] In the next few pages, I will try to outline some of the principles as well as the problems associated with marrow transplantation in man.

For purposes of clarity in later discussions, it is useful to view the interactions of the hematopoietic and lymphoid system in a somewhat oversimplified way. [5-7] In the marrow are pleuropotential stem cells (P cells) that may give rise to hematopoietic stem cells (H cells) or lymphcid stem cells (L cells). H cells leave the marrow via the blood to reside in the spleen and occasionally the liver. These cells, under the appropriate stimulus (primarily in the marrow), will differentiate into the more specialized granulocytes, erythrocytes and megakaryocytes.

The L cells may become bone marrow–derived lymphocytes, the so-called B lymphocyte, under the still undefined bursal equivalent in mammals. The B lymphocyte is highly specialized for eventual humoral

Supported in part by a grant CA-06973 from the National Cancer Institute and contract PH 43-66-924 from the National Institute of Allergy and Infectious Diseases.

Presented at the Symposium on Hematopoietic Stem Cells held at the Fifty-Fifth Annual Meeting of the Federation of the American Societies for Experimental Biology, Chicago, Ill, April 14, 1971.

antibody production requiring or not requiring the cooperation of a thymus-derived lymphocyte (depending upon the antigen). Some of these B cells migrate directly to the spleen, lymph node and peritoneal cavity. In the lymphatic tissues, the B lymphocyte, which is short-lived compared to the thymus-derived lymphocyte, occupies the outer cortex and medulla of lymph nodes as well as the periphery of spleen follicles and germinal centers.

The L cell may also migrate to the thymus or come under its hormonal influence to differentiate into a thymus-derived lymphocyte or T lymphocyte. The T lymphocyte will also migrate to the peripheral lymphatic tissues as well as return to the marrow. The T lymphocytes come to occupy the paracortical regions of the lymph nodes and periarteriolar areas of the spleen follicles and comprise a highly mobile population found in high concentration in the thoracic duct, lymph and peripheral blood. The T lymphocytes constitute the long-lived population and the cells of immunologic memory. Apart from its role in the cooperation with the B lymphocyte for certain types of humoral responses, it appears to be the cell involved in expressing cellular immunity.

The most logical application of marrow grafts would seem to be in those situations where there is failure of the P, H or L cells to perform their function either because of "experiments of nature" or because of external factors often created by man himself. One must recognize, however, the concept of at least two possibilities whenever a clinical situation appears wherein there appears to be a functional defect related to the marrow. Is the functional defect in question due to a failure of the microenvironment or is it due to an actual defect in the cell itself? Marrow transplantation is logical in the latter situation but not in the former.

Marrow transplantation has potential application in preparing individuals for organ grafting from the same donor and application in the treatment of certain forms of malignancy. The rationale for these approaches will be discussed below.

Failure of the Pleuropotential Cell (P Cell)

No proven examples exist of failure of the P cell in animal models or in human disease. Indeed, such conditions, if they do occur, are probably incompatible with life. There is a condition, however, where infants born with a form of lymphopenic thymic dysplasia have an additional defect, aleukocytosis. This condition has been termed reticular dysgenesis.[8,9] Because these children died in the first days of life, it has not been possible to obtain adequate information about their

73

hematopoietic and lymphoid systems. Morphologically, these children are extremely deficient. It has been suggested that this disorder involves a failure of the P cell to differentiate toward the H and L cell lines.[10] If the suggestion is true, we still have the question of whether or not we are dealing with a true cellular defect or a defect in the microenvironment. A marrow transplant in this situation might well clarify this issue.

Failure of the Immune System (L Cell)

Thymectomy in the newborn mouse has profound effects on the development of the immune system. In this situation, the absence of the appropriate microenvironment (thymus) precludes the continued development of T lymphocytes. Neither thymus extracts nor thymus cell suspensions can completely restore neonatally thymectomized animals to normal immunologic reactivity. If such mice are grafted with intact thymus tissue, however, they enjoy a normal life span, normally developed lymphoid tissues, and normal immune mechanisms. In such situations, most of the lymphoid cells multiplying in the spleen and thymus implant are of host (not donor) origin.[11] This latter observation and the requirements of an intact thymus structure lend support to the notion that it is the epithelial structures of the thymus that provide the necessary microenviornment for the development of the T lymphocyte.

The neonatally thymectomized mouse may represent a model for the clinical entity, congenital absence of the thymus and parathyroid glands with aortic arch anomaly, as described by DiGeorge.[12] Children with this apparently nonheritable syndrome fail to show any evidence of cellular immunity. They fail to show skin reactivity to a variety of bacterial, fungal and viral antigens. Delayed hypersensitivity to skin sensitizers cannot be induced in them. Furthermore, their lymphocytes fail to respond to PHA in culture and allogeneic skin grafts are not rejected.[12]

Thymic rather than marrow transplants would seem to be quite logical in this condition. In two instances where this has been attempted, delayed hypersensitivity and lymphocyte transformability were rapidly restored.[13,14] In both instances, theoretic and practical problems were encountered. Nevertheless, these initial attempts were encouraging. Donor-type lymphocytes were not found in the blood of these patients after thymic transplantation, which, of course, was to be expected from the experimental work of Miller.[11] It is interesting to speculate whether or not sufficient numbers of T lymphocytes might be transplanted with marrow in the human to repair, at least temporarily, the immunologic defect in DiGeorge syndrome. A marrow transplant would not seem to hold any advantage over a thymic implant except that of ease of procurement. On the other hand, the risk of graft-versus-host disease (GVH) would seem to be greater with a marrow transplant as opposed to a thymic implant.[15]

There are certain immune-deficiency syndromes with no demonstrable ability to make antibody or express cell-mediated immune reactions, with varying degrees of lymphopenia and different modes of inheritance.[16] It has been suggested that some of these diseases arise from a primary inability of in the P cell to differentiate into the L cell or in a primary defect in the L cell itself.[10] Indeed, a therapeutic effect has been seen with marrow grafts from histocompatible siblings.[17-20] One of the reported cases was the sex-linked form of lymphopenic hypogammaglobulinemia [19] and two were the autosomal form (Swiss-type).[18,20]

There are a number of other immunologic deficiency diseases that may be related to failure of a differentiative pathway of the L cell because of a cellular or microenvironment defect. Unfortunately, however, the description, classification and understanding of these diseases are still far from complete.[21] Nevertheless, marrow transplantation has been attempted in two of these disease syndromes.

The Wiskott-Aldrich syndrome (sex-linked recessive) is characterized by recurrent pyogenic infections, eczema and thrombocytopenia.[22,23] There is lymphopenia, lack of delayed hypersensitivity as assayed by skin tests and defective lymphocyte blastogenesis *in vitro* in response to PHA and to specific antigens.[24] These patients also have a defective humoral antibody response to carbohydrate but not to protein antigen.[25] The lack of antibodies to carbohydrate antigens is thought to be due to a failure to process the antigen, presumably by macrophages.[25]

Bach et al[26] transplanted marrow to a patient with the Wiskott-Aldrich syndrome. The donor was a HL-A matched sibling and the patient was prepared with immunosuppressive, employing the alkylating agent cyclophosphamide (CY) as outlined by Santos et al.[27] The patient experienced a dramatic clinical improvement and remained well for at least 24 months thereafter. Platelet levels, however, did not increase markedly and marrow karyotypes were recipient cell in type. Karyotype analysis of the blood revealed a relatively stable population of donor-type lymphocytes (about 20%).[28] A number of questions are raised by this case. By what mechanism was this patient improved? Was it due in part to transfer factor [29] that has been reported at least partially to repair this condition [30] or was it due to the few donor lymphocytes that enjoyed a long-term engraftment?.

Mucocutaneous candidiasis is a chronic infection by *Candida albicans* involving the skin, nails, scalp and vaginal and buccal mucous membranes.[31] Many patients with this disease fail to exhibit cutaneous cellular hypersensitivity to the causative organism although they are capable of specific immunoglobulin production.[32,33] Lymphocytes from these patients are usually capable of blast transformation in response to PHA and in some cases to *Candida* antigen[34,35] even though these patients are unable to produce macrophage migration-inhibition factor (MIF, a mediator associated with delayed hypersensitivity after antigeneic challenge) or exhibit delayed hypersensitivity when skin-tested.

Buckley *et al*[36] reported immunologic reconstitution in a patient with chronic mucocutaneous candidiasis by means of a bone marrow transplant without preceeding immunosuppresive therapy. Delayed hypersensitivity to *Candida* and two other antigens was detected 6 months after the transplant and a good therapeutic result was said to have been obtained. There was no evidence in this case, however, for the take or persistance of the infused marrow cells. It would be tempting to ascribe the patient's improvement to transfer factor carried by the infused marrow cells since transfer factor has improved children with this disease.[37] This cannot be the entire explanation, however, since Buckley *et al*[38] were able to induce delayed hypersensitivity to a contact allergen after the transplant. Transfer factor can only transfer the delayed hypersensitivity of the donor and not the ability to be sensitized.[29]

Failure of the Hematopoietic System (H Cells)

Failure of the microenvironment may result from the lack of important local stromal factors as well as a more general deficiency of hormones, natural poietins or nutritional requirements. In the broadest sense, failure of the microenvironment would also include situations where noxious factors are operative, such as infectious agents, chemical agents, physical agents or immunologic factors operative in certain autoimmune conditions. Many of the causes of microenvironment failure have been known for some time and are trivial and easily correctable, while the cause of others have been more occult but nevertheless have been found after intensive and often brilliant investigation.

The concept of the stromal microenvironment determining hematopoietic differentiation has gained considerable support from studies of mice with mutations at the W and Sl loci.[39] Mice of genotype Sl/Sl^d or W/W^v are markedly anemic, have no pigment-producing cells in their skin and are sterile. The basis for these defects are different for each of the mutations. The W/W^v mice have defective hematopoietic stem cells[40] as well as defective pigment-producing cells.[41] In Sl/Sl^d mice there is a defect in the microenvironment that prevents hematopoiesis [42] and pigment production. In both conditions, the L cell and its microenvironment appear to be intact.[43]

The Sl/Sl^d mouse, as noted above, provides a relatively clear example of a situation in which the microenvironment for hematopoiesis is genetically defective while the H cell itself appears normal. Recently, it has been reported that such mice may be restored to normal by grafts of spleen stroma which are able to provide the proper microenvironment for normal hematopoiesis.[44] This latter observation is of great interest and offers therapeutic possibilities for the as yet to be discovered human counterpart of the Sl/Sl^d model.

The W/W^v mouse provides perhaps the best model of marrow failure due to an H cell defect.[39,40] Indeed, the defective hematopoiesis in these mice have been repaired by allogeneic marrow transplants after whole-body x-irradiation.[45]

Ionizing radiation as well as a variety of cytotoxic agents are capable of producing lethal effects by destroying or at least severely injuring the H cell. The transplantation of syngeneic marrow has effectively reversed these lethal effects in many instances.[2] In other situations, allogeneic marrow has also been able to reverse these effects occurring after x-ray [2] and the alkylating agents aminochlorambucil [46] and CY.[27,47,48] Although marrow infusions have successfully reversed potentially lethal doses of ionizing radiation in reactor accidents [49,50] or in therapeutic misadventure with cytotoxic agents,[46] the greatest incidence of potentially fatal aplasia is seen under conditions where aplasia is induced intentionally for the purposes of marrow grafting.

As was noted in preceeding discussion, a variety of chemical and physical agents may be causally related to aplasia. About 50% of all cases of aplasia have no known cause.[51] A priori in most of these situations, one does not know with any degree of certainty whether the persisting defect is in the microenvironment or in the H cell itself. Some insight into this question has been provided, however, by clinical studies wherein various forms of aplasia have been corrected by marrow infusions.

At least 10 patients with aplasia have received syngeneic (ie, identical twins) marrow transplants. Three died before the effect of the infusion could be evaluated and two were not benefited by the procedure. Five patients recovered completely and the time of recovery after infusion indicated successful marrow transplantation. Of the successful cases, 3 were idiopathic, 1 was after chloramphenicol and 1 after anticonvulsant drugs were administered.[52]

Amiel *et al* [53] reported successful partial but persistent allogeneic marrow takes that dramatically improved the clinical status of the patients in 1 case of idiopathic aplasia, 1 case after chloramphenicol and in 1 case after hepatitis. No evidence of a take was demonstrated in 4 other cases of idiopathic aplasia. Immunosuppression was provided by pretreatment with an antilymphocyte globulin fraction.

The results reported above are encouraging and clearly demonstrate that in some cases of aplasia, the microenvironment is able to support the proliferation and differentiation of H cells. The reported failures with allogeneic cells [3] do not rule out the possibility that a stem cell defect was operative since immunosuppression may not have been adequate in these patients, many of whom may have been presensitized to major or minor transplantation antigens of their donor because of preceding blood transfusions.

Fanconi's syndrome or congenital pancytopenia is a condition wherein there are varying degrees of pancytopenia as well as other congenital malformations. The etiology of the disorder is unknown but is generally believed to be hereditary, perhaps due to a recessive gene, or the result of reciprocal chromosomal translocation in one of the parents and a duplication deficiency in the affected offspring. Cytogenetic studies have revealed a variety of structural abberations and a specific type of polyploidy.[54] Although it is possible that this disease is due to an H cell defect, it is also possible that it may represent a failure of the complete hematopoietic environment. Marrow transplantation in this disease would undoubtedly yield interesting clues as to its true etiology.

Apart from disorders of the H cell itself, there may be cellular defects in the erythrocyte, granulocyte or megakaryocyte cell lines. In many instances, cellular defects are suspected as it is in the clinical hemaglobinopathies, congenital spherocytosis or in the flextail mutation in mice where the mutation affects differentiation of erythropoietic cells but has no effect on the production of granulocytes.[55] In a number of instances, however, the available evidence does not allow one to discriminate between cellular defects independent of the microenvironment or defects of the micoenvironment that may be private to a given line of differentiated hematopoietic cells. A condition has been described, for instance, of an anemic individual whose plasma contained no transferrin.[56] This person might have been classed as having a type of idiopathic anemia possibly related to a cellular defect in the erythrocyte series if levels of transferrin not been determined. It is interesting to speculate that a marrow graft nevertheless may have repaired the anemia since cells derived from marrow infusions are capable of producing transferrin.[57]

In principle, it would seem logical to attempt marrow transplantation in the more severe forms of the hemoglobinopathies such as sickle cell anemia and certain types of the thalassemias. Except for a few unsuccessful attempts recently,[4] transplantation for these disorders has not been used in the past. Although these diseases may be servere, the prognosis is much better than that of aplastic anemia, acute leukemia and some of the immunologic deficiency diseases. Success with marrow transplantation in these latter areas undoubtedly will lead to an increase in therapeutic trials in sickle cell anemia and thalassemia.

Marrow Transplantation as a Prelude to Organ Grafting

The successful transplantation of allogeneic or even xenogeneic marrow allows the permanent survival of other tissue grafts from the same donor[58] or in the case of inbred animals from the same inbred strain.[2] Rats[47] and mice[48] given allogeneic marrow or lymphohematopoietic cells after CY treatment will accept both host- and donor-type skin while rejecting third-party skin. Such animals will also accept host-type kidney grafts.[59] Indeed, mice given rat bone marrow after lethal irradiation will accept subcutaneously placed grafts of rat pulmonary tissue.[60] At the present time, however, this offers only a hope for the future use in the clinic because of the as yet unresolved hazards associated with marrow transplants in man.

Use of Marrow Grafts in Malignancy

There are at least three reasons why one might wish to employ marrow transplantation in malignancy: (1) to provide the means of administering doses of anticancer agents in what would ordinarily be lethal doses were it not for the protection afforded by transplanted marrow; (2) to provide specific immunotherapy by the transplantation of syngeneic marrow and (3) to provide a therapeutic effect by means of a mild or controlled GVH utilizing allogeneic marrow.

For purposes of discussion, it is useful to consider that tumor cells may offer normal as well as tumor-specific transplantation antigens as two potential targets for reactive lymphoid cells or cytotoxic antibody. Lymphoid-derived and leukemic tumor cells are relatively rich in normal transplantation antigens while nonlymphoid-derived tumors such as fibrosarcoma and adenocarcinoma tumors may be relatively poor in such antigens. On the other hand, the strength of tumor-specific transplantation antigens will vary from tumor to tumor.

The infusion of syngeneic marrow after x-irradiation or chemotherapy in animals has generally been disappointing particularly in situations where tumor-specific antigens are weak or in doubt.[2] A similar failure of this approach to show a marked effect in the clinic has been reported by Thomas et al,[50] who reported on 3 patients with acute leukemia who were given 800–1000 rads whole-body x-irradiation and then marrow from an identical twin. These patients recovered from the irradiation but leukemia recurred 48–84 days later. A fourth patient was given 1596 rads and syngeneic marrow and showed hematopoietic recovery but died early after the transplant of hepatic failure, presumably due to viral hepatitis.

In situations where strong tumor-specific transplantation antigens were present or suspected in rodents, lethal x-irradiation or chemotherapy followed by syngeneic marrow and lymphoid cells has occasionally had remarkable therapeutic results,[2] but has often been without therapeutic benefit.[61-63] In experiments where an antigenic tumor was treated with a nonimmunosuppressive agent (dimethyl myleran), a marked therapeutic effect was seen.[61] The success of therapy apparently depended upon the synergism between the antitumor action of the drug and the immunologic resistance of the host to tumor-specific transplantation antigens.

Another approach has been to employ syngeneic lymphohematopoietic cells sensitized to putative tumor antigens. This form of immunotherapy has been reported to be successful even against established clinically detectable primary tumors induced by Moloney sarcoma virus.[63] In addition, an additive therapeutic effect of CY treatment given prior to sensitized syngeneic cells has been reported.[63]

Identical twin human donors have not been immunized with putative tumor antigens for obvious ethical reasons. Thomas et al,[50] however, have employed a unique approach. They treated 3 patients with leukemia and one with lymphosarcoma with whole-body x-irradiation followed by syngeneic marrow transplants and subsequent buffy coat cells from the donors. The patients were then given weekly subcutaneous injections of previously stored but irradiated tumor cells in an attempt to immunize donor cells. Two patients relapsed with leukemia, one 33 days and the other 8 months later. Another died of intersitital pneumonitis, without leukemia. The patient with lymphosarcoma was in complete remission 105 days post-transplant at the time of the report. The effectiveness of this novel approach can only be judged after further trials.

Lethal doses of whole-body x-irradiation [2] or high but nonlethal doses of CY [62] followed by allogeneic bone marrow and lymphoid cells have been shown in many cases to give a marked antitumor effect and have

80

even resulted in the total eradication of leukemic or lymphoid-derived tumors in animal systems. A few animals were able to survive free of tumor[2] but the majority died of GVH. Effective treatment of GVH disease increased the number of tumor-free survivors.[62,64]

In at least two reports, it was noted that severe GVH was without effect on a fibrosarcoma and adenocarcinoma in the mouse.[63,65] It has been suggested that the difference in results with lymphomas and leukemias on the one hand and these nonlymphomatous solid tumors on the other is a reflection of the relative richness of transplantation antigens on the surface of lymphoid and leukemic tumor cells (increased sensitivity to GVH) as opposed to other tumors.[65] In one case of a viral-induced fibrosarcoma in mice, the use of allogeneic cells presensitized to tumor antigens was effective in eliminating tumor cells when administered after CY.[63]

In general, transplanting allogeneic non–HL-A identical marrow in human leukemia after lethal doses of x-ray or CY has either failed to show takes or has resulted in death from GVH.[2,3,66] The one exception is a case of acute lymphocytic leukemia reported by Mathe et al.[58] The patient survived free of leukemia for 20 months after a lethal dose of x-ray and marrow infusion, but he died of a generalized herpes infection.

The major transplantation antigens in man are controlled by genes at one chromosmal locus designated HL-A.[67] Genetic analysis of family typing data permits the recognition of allogeneic siblings who are identical for both parental alleles. For purposes of discussion, these donor-recipient pairs will be called HL-A identical sibling matches. Recently, a number of marrow transplants have been attempted in patients with acute leukemia or lymphoma after lethal whole-body irradiation or CY treatment, using HL-A identical sibling matches. The rationale and experimental data related to the use of CY for marrow transplantation in man has been developed previously.[27]

Santos et al[68] performed marrow grafts in 5 patients with acute myelocytic leukemia and in 1 with acute monocytic leukemia, using HL-A matched siblings. Patients were prepared with four daily doses of CY (50–60 mg/kg per dose) and all but 1 patient recieved additional CY after the grafting. One patient, who may have been presensitized to donor antigens, did not show evidence of engraftment but did enjoy a remission of his disease before relapse 3 months later. Prompt marrow engraftment was seen in the other 4 patients who had donors of the opposite sex. During the first 30 days after transplant, both host- and donor-type cells were seen on karyotype analysis. Subsequently, however, only donor-type cells were seen. Two patients died of bacterial sepsis, one at 32 days and the other at 47 days after transplant. One patient died of GVH with terminal generalized viral infection 75 days after transplant and 1 patient died of acute staphylococcal pneumonitis 215 days after transplant. None of the 4 patients with marrow engraftment showed evidence of leukemia at autopsy.

Graw et al[69] performed marrow grafts with HL-A matched siblings in 7 patients with acute lymphocytic leukemia. A CY schedule designed after that described by Santos et al[27] was used in five instances but the dose was lower (45 mg/kg for each of 4 successive days) and whole-body x-ray was used in 2 patients. One patient failed to show a take (there was a major blood group mismatch) but prompt evidence of engraftment occurred in the other 6. One of the patients treated with x-ray failed to show a graft and the other died of GVH. Patients treated with CY never demonstrated complete chimerism[70] (ie, host-type lymphohematopoietic cells were present in all analyses) and acute leukemia recurred in all but 1 who died of GVH. Where testable by karyotype analysis, the recurrent leukemia was shown to be of host origin.[70] The recurrence of leukemia in these cases may possibly be related to the failure of these workers to obtain "complete" chimerism. It is most likely that the doses of CY were too low in these cases as contrasted to the higher doses employed by Santos et al.[68] Experiments in a rodent model reported elsewhere add credence to this suggestion.[47]

Thomas et al[71] treated 6 patients with acute leukemia and one with Hodgkin's disease with 1000 rads of whole-body x-irradiation, then with marrow from HL-A matched siblings and subsequently administered methotrexate to control GVH. The patient with Hodgkin's disease died of GVH but free of tumor at autopsy 37 days after transplant. Three patients died without evidence of a take. Two patients showed prompt marrow engraftment but relapsed with leukemia. One patient has a complete graft and is free of leukemia 200 days post-transplant.[72] In one of the cases of leukemia recurrence in a female, the leukemic cells were shown to possess the male karyotype of the donor.[73] The latter observation obviously suggests that an oncogenic virus was involved. Recent observations such as those of Brockman et al[74] show that the streptovaricins inhibit RNA-dependent DNA polymerase present in an oncogenic RNA virus and offer the hope for the future that such compounds might be administered after transplantation to prevent the transformation of donor cells by possible oncogenic viruses.

GVH Disease

GVH has been encountered in several situations in which individuals have been unable to defend themselves against grafts of immunologically competent allogeneic cells either because of immunoincompetence produced by disease states [16] or because of immunosuppressive treatment.[2] The clinical and pathologic aspects of this disease in animals and man have been extensively reviewed elsewhere.[2] In animals, CY,[2,75] methotrexate [2,76] and antilymphocyte sera [2,77] have been successful in controlling the severity of GHV. In addition, fractionation of marrow has also been shown to be effective.[78]

In man, there have not been enough clinical trials to indicate which of the above methods might be employed to successfully control severe GVH. The results of administering CY and methotrexate after transplantation of HL-A matched sibling transplants, however, has been encouraging. Of 16 such marrow transplants performed by the groups at Johns Hopkins University[68] the University of Washington [71] and the National Cancer Institute,[69] where there was evidence of engraftment, mild (transient skin rash) or no GVH was seen in 6 patients. Moderately severe GVH with definite skin involvement and occasional abnormalities in liver function was seen in 5. Severe GVH that led to death occurred in 5. It is of interest that 3 of the 5 patients with severe GVH either did not receive after the transplant CY or methotrexate (as is the present practice of the 3 groups) or were given unirradiated lymphocytes contaminating platelet donations (a situation known to increase the severity of GHV).

Conclusions

The rationale for and some of the results of marrow transplantation in human disease have been outlined. There have been a few notable successes but the majority of clinical attempts have failed. Nevertheless, the information gained in the practical and theoretic spheres suggests optimism for the future of this procedure. Continued animal and clinical research centered on the control of GVH, prevention of oncogenic viral transformation and the supportive care of individuals during periods of aplasia hopefully will justify the present optimism.

References

1. Jacobson LO, Marks EK, Robson, MJ, Gaston EO, Zirkle RE: Effect of spleen protection on mortality following X-irradiation. J Lab Clin Med 34:1538–1543, 1949
2. van Bekkum DW, deVries MJ: Radiation Chimeras. London, Logos Press, 1967, pp 1–277
3. Bortin M: A compendium of reported human bone marrow transplants. Transplantation 9:571–587, 1970

4. Congdon CC: Cooperative group on bone marrow transplantation in man: report of work sessions held June 16–17, 1969, at Hôpital Paul-Brousse, Villejuif, France. Exp Hematol 20:97–116, 1970

5. Cooper MD, Perey DY, Peterson RDA, Gabrielsen AE, Good RA: The two-component concept of the lymphoid system, Immunologic Deficiency Diseases in Man. Edited by D Bergsma, RA Good. New York, The National Foundation–March of Dimes, 1967, pp 7–12

6. Good RA, Peterson RDA Perey DY, Finstad J, Cooper MD:[5] pp 17–34

7. Antigen Sensitive Cells. Edited by G Möller. Transplant Rev 1:1–149, 1969

8. deVaal OM, Seynhaeve V: Reticular dysgenesia. Lancet 2:1123–25, 1959

9. Gitlin D, Vawter G, Craig JM: Thymic alymphoplasia and congenital aleukocytosis. Pediatrics 33:184–192, 1964

10. Hoyer JR, Cooper MD, Gabrielsen AE, Good RA: Lymphopenic forms of congenital immunological deficiency: clinical and pathological patterns,[5] pp 91–103

11. Miller JFAP: Effect of thymic ablation and replacement, The Thymus in Immunology. Edited by RA Good, AE Gabrielsen, New York, Harper & Row, Publishers, 1964, pp 436–464

12. DiGeorge AM: Congenital absence of the thymus and its immunologic consequences: concurrence with congenital hypoparathyroidism.[5] pp 116–121

13. August CS, Rosen FS, Filler RM, Janeway CA, Markowski B, Kay HEM: Implantation of a fetal thymus restoring immunological competence in a patient with thymic aplasia (DiGeorge's syndrome). Lancet 2:1210–1211, 1968

14. Cleveland WW, Fogel BJ, Brown WT, Kay HEM: Fetal thymic transplant in a case of DiGeorge's syndrome. Lancet 2:1211–1214, 1968

15. Owens AH Jr, Santos GW: The induction of graft versus host disease in mice treated with cyclophosphamide. J Exp Med 128:277–291, 1968

16. Immunologic Deficiency Diseases in Man. Edited by D Bergsma and RA Good. New York, The National Foundation–March of Dimes, 1967, pp 1–473

17. Hitzig WH, Willi H: Hereditare lymphoplasmocytare dystenesie ("Alymphocytose mit agammeglobulinamie"). Schweiz Med Wochenschr 91:1625–1633, 1961

18. Meuwissen HJ, Rodey G, McArthur J, Pabst H, Gatti R, Chilgren R, Hong R, Frommel D, Coifman R, Good RA: Bone marrow transplantation: therapeutic usefulness and complications. Am J Med 51:513–532, 1971

19. Meuwissen HJ, Gatti RA, Terasaki PI, Hong R, Good RA: Treatment of lymphopenic hypogammaglobulinemia and bone marrow aplasia by transplantation of allogeneic marrow. N Engl J Med 281:691–697, 1969

20. DeKoning J, Dooren LJ, van Bekkum DW, van Rood JJ, Dicke KA, Radl, J: Transplantation of bone marrow cells and fetal thymus in an infant with lymphopenic immunological deficiency. Lancet 1:1223–1227, 1969

21. Kay HEM: States of immune deficiency (Editorial). Rev Europ D'Etudes Clin Biol 15:249–252, 1970

22. Wiskott A: Familiärer, angeborener, morbus warlhoffi? Monatsschr Kinderheilk 68:212–216, 1937

23. Aldrich RA, Steinberg AC, Campbell DC: Pedigree demonstrating a sex-linked recessive condition characterized by draining ears, eczematoid dermatitis and bloody diarrhea. Pediatrics 13:133–139, 1954

84

24. Oppenheim JJ, Blaese RM, Waldman, TA: Defective lymphocyte transformation and delayed hypersensitivity in Wiskott-Aldrich syndrome. J Immunol 104:835–844, 1970

25. Cooper MD, Chase HP, Lowman JT, Krivit W, Good RA: Wiskott-Aldrich syndrome: an immunologic deficiency disease involving the afferent limb of immunity. Am J Med 44:499–513, 1968

26. Bach FH, Joo P, Albertini RJ, Anderson JL, Borton MM: Bone marrow transplantation in a patient with Wiskott-Aldrich syndrome. Lancet 2:1364–1366, 1968

27. Santos GW, Burke PJ, Sensenbrenner LL, Owens AH Jr: Rationale for the use of cyclophosphamide as immunosuppression for marrow transplants in man. International Symposium on Pharmacologic Treatment in Organ and Tissue Transplantation, Milan, Italy, 1969. Edited by A Bertelli and AP Monaco, pp 24–31

28. Bach FH: Personal communication

29. Lawrence HS, Valentine FT: Transfer factor and other mediators of cellular immunity. Am J Pathol 60:437–451, 1970

30. Levin AS, Spitler LE, Stites DP, Fudenberg HH: Wiskott-Aldrich syndrome, a genetically determined cellular immunologic deficiency: Clinical and laboratory responses to therapy with transfer factor. Proc Natl Acad Sci USA 67:821–828, 1970

31. Winner HL, Hurley R: Candida Albicans. Boston, Little Brown and Company, 1964, pp 1–306

32. Chilgren RS, Meuwissen HJ, Quie PG, Hong R: Chronic mucocutaneous candidiasis, deficiency of delayed hypersensitivity and selective local antibody defect. Lancet 2:688–693, 1967

33. Imperato PJ, Buckley CE III, Callaway JL: Candida granuloma: a clinical and immunology study. Arch Dermatol 97:139–146, 1968

34. Chilgren RS, Meuwissen HJ, Quie PG, Good RA, Hong R: The cellular immune defect in chronic mucocutaneous candidiasis. Lancet 1:1286–1288, 1969

35. Marmor ME, Barnett EV: Cutaneous anergy without systemic disease: a syndrome associated with mucocutaneous fungal infection. Am J Med 44:979–989, 1968

36. Buckley RH, Lucas ZJ, Hattler BG Jr, Zmijewski, CM, Amos DB: Defective cellular immunity associated with chronic mucocutaneous moniliasis and recurrent staphylococcal botryomycosis: immunological reconstitution by allogeneic bone marrow. Clin Exp Immunol 3:153–169, 1968

37. Rocklin RE, Chilgren RA, Hong R, David JR: Transfer of cellular hypersensitivity in chronic mucocutaneous candidiasis monitored *in vivo* and *in vitro*. Cell Immunol 1:290–299, 1970

38. Buckley RH: Personal communication.

39. Russell ES: Problems and potentialities in the study of genic action in the mouse, Methodology in Mammalian Genetics, Edited by WJ Burdette. San Francisco, Holden-Day Inc, 1963, pp 217–232

40. McCulloch EA, Siminovitch L, Till JE: Spleen colony formation in anemia mice of genotype W/W^v. Science 144:844–845, 1964

41. Mayer TG, Green MC: An experimental analysis of the pigment defect caused by mutations at the W and Sl loci in mice. Dev Biol 18:62–75, 1968

42. McCulloch EA, Siminovitch L, Till JE, Russell ES, Bernstein SE: The

cellular basis of the genetically determined hematopoietic defect in anemia mice of genotype Sl/Sl^d. Blood 26:399–410, 1965

43. Mekori T, Phillips RA: The immune response in mice of genotypes W/W^v and Sl/Sl^d. Proc Soc Expt Biol Med 132:115–119, 1969
44. Bernstein SF: Tissue transplantation as an analytic and therapeutic tool in hereditary anemias. Am J Surg 119:448–451, 1970
45. Russell ES, Smith LJ, Lawson FA: Implantation of normal blood forming tissue in radiated genetically anemic hosts. Science 124:1076–1077, 1956
46. Beilby JOW, Cade IS, Jellife AM, Parkin DM, Stewart JW: Prolonged survival of a bone marrow graft resulting in a blood-group chimera. Br Med J 1:96–99, 1960
47. Santos GW, Owens AH Jr: Syngeneic and allogeneic marrow transplants in the cyclophosphamide pretreated rat, Advance in Transplantation. Edited by J Dausset, J Hamburger, G Mathe. Copenhagen, Munksgaard, 1968, pp 431–436
48. Santos GW, Owens AH Jr: Allogeneic marrow transplantation in cyclophosphamide-treated mice. Transpl Proc 1:44–46, 1969
49. Jammet H, Mathé G, Pendic B, Duplan JF, Maupin B, Latarjet R, Kalic D, Schwartzenberg L, Djukic Z, Vigne J: Etude de six cas d'irradiation total aiguë accidentelle. Rev Fr Etudes Clin Biol 4:210–225, 1959
50. Thomas ED, Rudolph RH, Fefer A, Storb R, Slichter S Buckner CD: Isogeneic marrow grafting in man. Exp Hematol 21:16–18, 1971
51. Scott JL, Cartwright GE, Wintrobe MM: Acquired aplastic anemia: an analysis of thirty-nine cases and review of the pertinent literature. Medicine 38:119–172, 1959
52. Pillow RP, Epstein RB, Buckner CD, Giblett ER, Thomas ED: Treatment of bone marrow failure by isogeneic marrow infusion. N Engl J Med 275:94–97, 1966
53. Amiel JF, Mathé G, Schwarzenberg L, Schneider M, Choay J, Trolard P, Hayat M, Schlumberger JR, Jasmin C: Les greffes de moelle osseuse allogénique après conditionnement par le seul sérum antilymphocytaire dans les états d'aplasie médullaire. Presse Med 78:1727–1734, 1970
54. Wintrobe MM: Clinical Hematology. Sixth edition. Philadelphia, Lea and Febiger, 1967, pp 795–796
55. Thompson MW, McCulloch EA, Siminovitch L, Till JE: The cellular basis for the defect in haemopoiesis in flexed-tail mice. I. Nature and persistence of the defect. Br J Haematol 12:152–160, 1966
56. Heilmeyer L: Die Atransferrinämien. Acta Haematol 36:40–49, 1966
57. Phillips ME, Thorbecke GJ: Studies on the serum proteins of chimeras. I. Identification and study of the site of origin of donor type serum proteins in adult rat into mouse chimeras. Int Arch Allergy 29:553–567, 1966
58. Mathé G, Amiel JL, Schwarzenberg L, Cattan A, Schneider M: Hematopoietic chimera in man after allogeneic (homologous) bone marrow transplantation: control of the secondary syndrome. Br Med J 2:1633–1635, 1963
59. Guttman RD, Santos GW, Lindquist RR: Unpublished observations
60. Santos GW, Garver RM, Cole LJ: Acceptance of rat and mouse lung grafts by radiation chimeras. J Natl Cancer Inst 24:1367–1387, 1960
61. Floersheim GL: Treatment of Moloney lymphoma with lethal doses of dimethyl-myleran combined with injections of haemopoietic cells. Lancet 1:228–233, 1969

62. Owens AH Jr: Effect of graft versus host disease on the course of L1210 leukemia. Exp Hematol 20:43–44, 1970

63. Fefer A: Immunotherapy of primary Moloney sarcoma virus-induced tumors. Int J Cancer 5:327–337, 1970

64. Boranić M: Transient graft versus host reaction in the treatment of leukemia in mice. J Natl Cancer Inst 41:421–437, 1968

65. Santos GW: Effect of graft versus host disease on a spontaneous adenocarcinoma in mice. Exp Hematol 20:46–48, 1970

66. Mathé G: Bone marrow transplantation, Human Transplantation. Edited by FT Rapaport, J Dausset. New York, Grune and Stratton, 1968, pp 284–303

67. Bach FH: Transplantation: pairing of donor and recipient. Science 168:1170–1179, 1970

68. Santos GW, Sensenbrenner LL, Burke PJ, Colvin OM, Owens AH Jr, Bias WB, Slavin RE: Marrow transplantation in man following cyclophosphamide. Transpl Proc 3:400–404, 1971

69. Graw RG, Leventhal BG, Yankee RA, Rogentine GN, Whang-Peng J, Herzig GP, Halterman RH, Henderson ES: HL-A and mixed leukocyte culture matched allogeneic bone marrow transplantation in patients with acute leukemia. Transpl Proc 3:405–408, 1971

70. Graw RG: Personal communication

71. Thomas ED, Bryant JI, Buckner CD, Chard RL, Clift RA, Epstein RB, Fefer A, Fialkow PJ, Funk DD, Giblett ER, Lerner KG, Neiman PE, Reynolds FA, Rudolph RH, Slichter S, Storb R: Allogeneic marrow grafting for hematologic malignancy. Blood 38:267–287, 1971

72. Thomas ED: Personal communication

73. Fialkow PJ, Thomas ED, Bryant JI, Neiman PE: Leukemic transformation of engrafted human marrow cells in vivo. Lancet 1:251–255, 1971

74. Brockman WW, Carter WA, Li HI, Reusser, F, Nichol FR: The streptovaricins inhibit RNA dependent DNA polymerase present in an oncogenic RNA virus. Nature 230:249–250, 1971

75. Owens AH Jr, Santos GW: The effect of cytotoxic drugs on graft versus host disease in mice. Transplantation 11:378–382, 1971

76. Storb R, Epstein RB, Graham TC, Thomas ED: Methotrexate regimens for control of graft versus host disease in dogs with allogeneic marrow grafts. Transplantation 9:240–246, 1970

77. Ledney GD: Antilymphocyte serum in the therapy and prevention of acute secondary disease in mice. Transplantation 8:127–140, 1969

78. Dicke KA, Tridente G, van Bekkum DW: The selective elimination of immunologically competent cells from bone marrow and lymphocyte cell mixtures. III. In vitro test for detection of immunocompetent cells in fractionated mouse spleen cell suspensions and primate bone marrow suspensions. Transplantation 8:422–434, 1969

The Use of Stem Cell Concentrates As Bone Marrow Grafts in Man

K. A. Dicke, U. W. Schaefer, and D. W. van Bekkum

IN humans, one of the severest complications of allogeneic bone marrow transplantation is the development of acute graft-versus-host (GVH) disease, 6–10 days after transplantation. This is due to an immunologic reaction against the host by the grafted immunocompetent cells (ICC), which cell type is present in a high proportion in primate bone marrow. One approach to mitigate acute GVH was recently introduced by our group, and consists of the separation between ICC and hemopoietic stem cells (HSC) by discontinuous albumin density centrifugation of the bone marrow cell suspension. The method was developed in mice, using spleen cells, because this cell population resembles primate bone marrow in its ICC/HSC ratio. In the mouse, quantitative evaluation of HSC and ICC was performed by the CFU-S[1] and the Simonsen assay,[2] respectively. In the monkey, an animal used for preclinical studies, the number of HSC and ICC in bone marrow fractions could not be estimated, since in vivo assays, as in the mouse, are not available. Therefore, it was necessary to develop quantitative methods for both cell types. At present, in vitro assays are available, the PHA response test for lymphocytes[3] and the agar colony formation assay for HSC.[4] Although the nature of the in vitro colony forming cell

---

Supported in part by the commission of the European communities (EURATOM) Brussels, Belgium, Contract 079-69-1 BIAC.

88

is still under dispute, we have obtained convincing evidence that the culture system we devised for this purpose does favor the production of colonies from pluripotent stem cells.[4] Using both in vitro methods as guides, the gradient method was adapted to separate monkey bone marrow suspensions. Similar in vitro assays have been developed in humans,[5] and by using these methods, a concentration of stem cells deprived of lymphocytes was shown in fraction 3 in gradients constituted on the basis of extrapolation from other species. Because of the limited yield of purified stem cells—10–20% of the number of HSC present in the original marrow suspension—clinical application of the technique has so far been restricted to patients requiring small bone marrow grafts, i.e., babies suffering from Combined Immune Deficiency Disease (CID). This disorder appears to be due to a defect in the pluripotent HSC in bone marrow.[6] Grafting lymphocyte-free HSC concentrates obtained by bone marrow fractionation of HL-A-identical donors appeared to be highly successful in curing the CID.[7,8]

Attempts were also undertaken to restore immunity by using lymphocyte-free marrow suspensions from HL-A-nonidentical donors. This step was important, since the availability of HL-A-identical donors is especially when unfractionated bone marfrom nonidentical donors carries a very high risk of fatal acute GVH, and, accordingly, one of us[9] had recommended that very small bone marrow grafts be used, especially when unfactionated bone marrow should be employed. In case such a graft fails to induce immune restoration as well as acute GVH, it seems justified to repeat that attempt with a slightly larger number of cells, an approach which has been called "sneak-in." The success of this sneak-in therapy can obviously be improved by grafting lymphocyte-poor HSC concentrates. However the low recovery of purified stem cells in the density gradient allowed one small graft, whereas second and even third transplants with increased cell numbers could hardly be carried out when the donor was a child from whom relatively small numbers of cells can be collected. Therefore, it was essential to improve the recovery of stem cells in the lymphocyte-poor fractions of the gradient. Another useful advice is the recent development of a storage technique, by Schaefer et al.,[10] which preserves stem-cell viability completely. This preservation technique allows one stem-cell concentrate to be used repeatedly, provided sufficiently large cell numbers can be obtained from the donor.

MODIFICATION OF THE HUMAN MARROW GRADIENT; THE USE OF STORED LARGE HSC GRAFTS

Technical details of the discontinuous albumin density gradient centrifugation technique have been described elsewhere,[3] and therefore the most important modifications only are mentioned here. It was known from data obtained in other species that slight changes in osmolarity of the albumin (bovine serum albumin) stock solution, from which the gradient is prepared, influence the separation of HSC and lymphocytes. In previous studies with human bone marrow, gradients were prepared from a stock solution of 375 mOsm. A decrease of 15 mOsm resulted in a gradient which yields a fraction 3 containing 5%–8% of the cells and up to 50% of the HSC. However, the number of PHA-responsive cells in that fraction was still up to 5% of the total, which is unacceptably high. To eliminate these cells, fraction 3 was refractionated, using a gradient prepared from a

Table 1. Distribution of Human Marrow CFU-C and PHA Response CFU-S in the Discontinuous Gradient*

| | Hemopoietic Stem Cell Assay | | | PHA Response |
	Number of CFU-C Per 10^5 Cells Plated P. Fract. (Mean)	Conc. Factor	Yield Hem.§ Stem Cells	Conc. Factor‡
Total	100 (80– 120)	1	100	1
Fr. 3 (5–8%)||	700 (500– 900)	7	40–45	1
Fr. 3/2 (0.3–0.5%)†	4000 (3000–5000)	40	15–20	<0.1
Fr. 3/3 (1–1.5%)†	2000 (1600–2400)	20	20–35	<0.1
Fr. 3/4 (1–2%)†	200 (150– 250)	2	2–4	2

*Average of 5 different fractionations.
†Fractions obtained by refractionation of Fr. 3
‡Activity expressed per 10^5 cells of unfractionated suspension and each fraction, obtained by multi-plication of the conc. factor and the percentage cell yield per fraction.
§Expressed as a percentage of total.
||Cell yield per fraction expressed as a percentage of total.

stock solution of 370 mOsm. From the results in Table 1, it can be noticed that fraction 3/2 and 3/3 contained 15%–20% and 20%–25% respectively of HSC and greatly reduced numbers of lymphocytes. Therefore, both fractions are suitable for transplantation. Together, they contain up to 40% of the total number of HSC.

The improvement of stem-cell recovery in the gradient makes it possible to extend the application of the gradient procedure also to aplastic patients in whom large grafts are needed. It has already become feasible to use the gradient in this category in host-donor combinations when the body weight ratio is 1:1.5. Moreover, the recently developed storage technique allows sufficient numbers of HSC to be collected from one donor during several sessions by repeated marrow aspirations.

RESULTS WITH STEM CELL GRAFTS IN CID

So far, we have assisted in the transplantation of ten CID infants with small amounts of enriched stem-cell fractions prepared by our technique.[11] Because of early mortality (before day 21 after transplantation), the effectivity of lymphocyte-poor stem-cell fractions can be evaluated in six cases only (Table 2). Two of these (Cases 1 and 9) received enriched stem-cell fractions from an HL-A identical donor, which resulted in complete reconstitution without any signs of a GVH reaction in one patient and with a short and very mild skin rash in the other. Four infants received stem-cell fractions from nonidentical donors; none of them developed acute GVH disease as seen after unfractioned marrow is grafted. In one of these patients (No. 9), a temporary take was observed, and this patient is still alive more than 2 yr after

Table 2. Immune Deficient Babies Treated with Bone Marrow Stem Cell Fractions

	Number of Grafted Fraction 3 Cells/kg Body Weight	Residual Cellular Immunity of Recipient	Infection at Time of Grafting	HL-A Identity	Take	Survival Time
1. Leiden 1968	5×10^6	−	Present	Yes	+	$> 2^{1}/_{2}$ yr
2. Boston 1969	5×10^6	−	Present	Yes ?	+	19 days
3. Minnesota 1969	5×10^6	−	Present	No	+	45 days
4. Ulm 1969	5×10^6	+	Absent	No	+*	> 1 yr
5. Leiden 1970	5×10^6	−	Present	Yes ?	?	12 days
6. Paris 1970	5×10^6	?	Present	No	?	12 days
7. Zürich 1970	2×10^7	+	Present	No	?	6 days
8. Copenhagen 1971	2×10^6 and 5×10^6	−	Present	No	+	70/94 days†
9. Leiden 1971	5×10^6	−	Absent	Yes (uncle)	+?‡	> 7 mo
10. Utrecht 1971	2×10^6	−	Absent ?	No	+	51/96/141 days†

*Temporary.
†Days after each successive transplantation.
‡All markers identical.

grafting. In this case, the diagnosis CID is not certain so that a detailed discussion concerning the effect of the graft falls beyond the scope of this paper. The reasons for the lack of effective immune restoration in Patients 3, 8, and 10 who were treated with non—HL-A identical cells are obscure, although definite signs of a take were present. A moderate delayed GVH appeared approximately 1 mo after grafting in these patients, who died on day 45, 50, and 70, respectively, after transplantation. The reason for death is not certain, although it was likely due to the severe infections from which the children were suffering. These infections are caused by pathogenic colibacteria, probably of endgenous origin, by invasion through the intestinal tract wall. Therefore, in future cases the patient will have to be decontaminated bacteriologically, if possible. In germ-free mice grafted with allogeneic bone marrow after lethal whole body irradiation, mortality from delayed GVH does not occur,[12,13] even after these animals are conventionalized after a certain time interval. This latter phenomenon is an important additional argument in favor of decontaminating the CID recipient.

CONCLUSIONS

(1) Small grafts of lymphocyte-poor HSC concentrates from HL-A identical donors completely reconstitute immunity in CID.

(2) Separation of marrow by discontinuous density gradient centrifugation effectively prevents *acute* GVH disease, even in non-HL-A identical situations.

(3) Large stem-cell concentrates can be prepared and stored, without loss of viability, so that the 'sneak-in' method, consisting of repeated small stem-cell grafts, can

be performed by grafting cells from one single stem-cell fraction. Preservation allows one to wait for the results of the in vitro assay for ICC and HSC before the stem cell fraction is grafted. Moreover, it is possible to extend the gradient to aplastic patients in whom large grafts are needed.

4) In non-HL-A identical recipient-donor combinations, severe infections are the main complication during the post-transplantation period in which delayed GVH is present. Therefore bacteriologic decontamination is strongly recomended.

REFERENCES

1. Till, J. E., and McCulloch, E. A.: Radiation Res. 14:213, 1961.

2. Simonsen, M., and Jensen, E.: *In* Albert F., and Lejeune-Ledant, G. (Eds): Biological Problems of Grafting, Oxford, Blackwell, 1959, p. 214.

3. Dicke, K. A., Tridente, G., and Bekkum, D. W. van: Transplantation 8:422, 1969.

4. —, Platenburg, M. G. C. and Bekkum, D. W. van: Cell Tissue Kinet. 4:463, 1971.

5. —, Noord, M. J.: CIBA Foundation Symposium, London, 1972. (In press).

6. Vries, M. J. de, Dooren, L. J., and Cleton, F. J. Bekkum, D. W. Van, Rood, J. J. van Dicke, K.A., and Ràdl, J.: Birth Defects. 4:173, 1968.

7. Koning, J. de, Dooren, L. J.: The Lancet 1:1223, 1969.

8. Voosen, J. M., de, Bekkum, D. W. van, Dicke, K. A., Evsvoogel, J. J. van, Way, D. vander, and Dooren, L. J.: Clin. Exp. Immunol. (In press).

9. Bekkum, D. W. van: Transplant. Rev. 9:3, 1972.

10. Schaefer, U. W., Dicke, K. A., and Bekkum, D. W. van: Rev. Eur. Etud. Clin. Biol. 17:483, 1972.

11. Bekkum, D. W. van, and Dicke, K. A.: *In* Ontogeny of Acquired Immunity. A CIBA Foundation Symposium, 1972, p. 223.

12. Jones, M., Wilson, R., and Bealmear, P.M.: Radiation Res. 45:577, 1971.

13. Waay, D. van der: Unpublished data.

Aplastic Anemia Treated by Marrow Tansplantation

C. D. Buckner, R. A. Clift, A. Fefer, D. D. Funk, H. Glucksberg,
R. E. Ramberg, R. Storb, and E. D. Thomas

MARROW transplantation has long offered the hope of permanent correction of marrow failure, whether due to disease, drug reaction or to an unknown cause.[1] However, fulfillment of this hope has been limited to those few cases in which the patient had an identical twin to serve as a marrow donor.[2] We previously reported four cases of marrow failure prepared for marrow grafting by administering cyclophosphamide (CY) followed by marrow from a sibling donor.[3] In each instance, the sibling donor was shown to have inherited the same two HL-A haplotypes as the patient, and the match was confirmed by nonreactivity in a mixed leukocyte culture (MLC). This report describes an additional four patients treated identically and presents a follow-up of the original two survivors.

MATERIALS AND METHODS

Techniques used in this laboratory have been given in detail in publications describing the technique of marrow grafting,[4] the MLC test,[5] the general management of patients undergoing marrow engraftment,[6] and cytogenetic methods.[7] The CY (Cytoxan, Mead Johnson, Evansville, Indiana) was administered according to the regimen of Santos et al.[8] The day of marrow infusion

---

Supported by Grant CA 10895, Training Grant CA 05231 and Contract PH 43-67-1435 from the U.S. Public Health Service, and by American Cancer Society Grant CI-52.

was designated "day 0" and subsequent days were numbered from that point. After marrow grafting, all fresh blood products were irradiated with 1500 rad in vitro before administration. The methotrexate (MTX) regimen after grafting, occasionally modified by clinical events, was 10–20 mg/sq m on day 1 and 10 mg/sq m on days 3, 6, 11, and weekly thereafter for 100 days.[6,9] All transfusions before grafting were from random donors, except in Patient 4 who had one transfusion from his mother. Granulocyte transfusions, utilizing the NCI-IBM blood cell separator,[10] were administered daily after the first dose of CY until definite engraftment in six patients (Cases 2, 4–8). The granulocyte donor was usually a parent or sibling, with occasional augmentation by granulocytes from donors with chronic myelogenous leukemia.

Patients

Table 1 summarizes the clinical data on the eight patients. All had totally aplastic or severely hypoplastic marrows on examination of aspirated marrow and biopsy. All were males except Case 1; the age range was from 13–60. In five, the etiology of marrow failure was unknown, and in one it followed a 3-yr history of paroxysmal nocturnal hemoglobinuria (PNH). In two patients, the marrow failure was associated with hepatitis, as a concomitant event in Case 4 and after 3 mo in Case 6. All patients except Case 4 had received androgens for at least 6 wk without a response. Four patients were treated with prednisone. Granulocyte levels ranged from 0–345/cu mm. Platelet levels ranged from 2250–5700/cu mm when not maintained by platelet transfusions. All had received multiple red cell and platelet transfusions. Three patients were refractory to random platelets due to isoimmunization. All patients had had at least one episode of infection which was treated with antibiotics, and four had had at least one episode of septicemia. Six patients were receiving antibiotics at the time of admission.

RESULTS

Table 2 summarizes the transplantation data on these eight patients. Marrow cells, 12–24 $\times$ 10^9, were infused 36 hr after the last dose of CY, representing a marrow

97

Table 1. Clinical Details of Transplanted Patients

Case Number	Age (yr)	Etiology	Granulocyte Level (cumm)	Platelet Level (cumm)	Duration of Pancytopenia (mo)	RBC Transfusions (units)	Platelet Transfusions (units)	Refractory to Platelets
1	60	Idiopathic	345	4,800	12	18	8	Yes
2	16	Idiopathic	200	5,000	6	34	53	No
3	19	Idiopathic	0	5,000	7	39	19	No
4	13	Hepatitis	220	2,250	2	10	140	No
5	23	PNH	75	3,500	7	44	8	Yes
6	31	Hepatitis	0	5,700	2	4	26	Yes
7	41	Idiopathic	0	3,000	3	18	16	No
8	19	Idiopathic	0	3,000	2	17	43	No

Table 2. Results of Marrow Transplantation

Case Number	Marrow Cells Infused (10^8/kg)	Engraftment	GVH	Survival (Days)	Cause of Death
1	3.0	Yes	++++	45	GVH, Infection
2	1.7	Yes	0	>492	Living
3	2.0	Yes	0	67	Graft rejection, Infection
4	3.3	Yes	+	>415	Living
5	2.0	Yes	0	>310	Living
6	2.4	Yes	++++	85	GVH, Infection
7	2.0	Yes	0	>186	Living
8	4.0	No	0	0	Cardiac failure

dose of $1.7\text{--}4.0 \times 10^8$ marrow cells/kg body weight. Seven of eight patients achieved engraftment, as determined by a rise in peripheral blood counts after the post CY nadir. This was confirmed by cytogenetic analysis in the six patients who had donors of opposite sex and by a red cell marker in Case 7. All marrow and stimulated peripheral blood cytogenetic studies, up to the present time or at the time of death, showed only donor karyotypes, except Case 3. This patient achieved a prompt graft but rejected it. The rejection process began around day 36, with progression to total marrow failure. Cytogenetic studies on day 17 revealed all marrow cells were of donor origin. On day 40, host cells appeared in phytohemagglutinin-stimulated preparations of marrow and peripheral blood with subsequent total reversion to host-type cells.

Graft-versus—host disease (GVH) was definitely present in three patients (Cases 1, 3, and 6) and was fatal in two (Cases 1 and 6). The two patients who died developed skin rash, diarrhea, and progressive hepatic dysfunction, beginning in the fourth week post-transplant and leading to death due to infectious complications in 45 and 85 days. On day 19, Patient 4 developed a rash, which was characteristic of GVH clinically and on biopsy. Diarrhea and liver function abnormalities subsequently developed, but all signs and symptoms resolved by day 40.

Patients 2, 5, and 7 developed liver function abnormalities characteristic of active hepatitis during the first 3 mo after engraftment. Case 2 had a positive test for Australia antigen before admission, which has persisted to the present time. No definite etiology could be established in the other two patients, and there was complete resol-

Table 3. Hematologic Values in Surviving Patients

Case Number	Day	White Blood Cells (cumm)	Granulo-cytes (cumm)	Plate-lets (cumm)	Hemato-crit (Vol %)
2	442	6,900	3,000	340,000	40.0
4	379	3,700	1,800	242,000	36.0
5	204	8,300	4,100	163,000	42.0
7	151	10,000	3,800	257,000	38.0

ution in Cases 2 and 5, but Patient 7 had a persistently elevated SGOT and alkaline phosphatase at 194 days.

One patient (Case 8) died of intractable congestive heart failure on the day of marrow infusion. Creatine phosphokinase levels were not elevated during or after CY administration, although there was a progressive voltage decrease on EKG. At autopsy, the most prominent finding was pulmonary edema, but histologically there were no myocardial lesions.

Four patients are alive 186, 310, 415, and 492 days after engraftment, with normal marrow function (Table 3). Three patients have resumed normal activity. One patient (Case 7) has not resumed full activity and continues to have active hepatitis.

DISCUSSION

These results clearly demonstrate the feasibility of allogeneic marrow transplantation as a potentially curative technique in patients with total marrow failure. These data, in addition to previous results in the identical twin transplants,[2] indicate that the defect in aplastic anemia is usually a stem-cell abnormality and not a disease of the marrow microenvironment, as suggested by Knospe and Crosby.[11]

The long-term persistence of marrow function in four of eight patients with this degree of marrow faliure is encouraging, as none of these patients were expected to survive with supportive care alone. Three of the eight patients were completely unresponsibe to random platelet transfusions, and the remaining patients, if they had not died of infectious complications would have become immunized.[12] The only treatment for such patients is repeated transfusions from HL-A matched siblings.[12] There is some indication that such long-term platelet support is feasible, but it puts a large burden on the donor.[12] In addition, the possibility of immunization against a future transplant by transfusing HL-A compatible blood products has been clearly demonstrated in the dog,[13] so that platelet support from an HL-A-matched sibling may significantly decrease the chances of a successful transplant. One patient in this series underwent graft rejection, possibly as a consequence of immunization to non-HL-A antigens by prior transfusion. At the present time this phenomenon cannot be predicted or prevented.

Two patients in this series developed fatal GVH disease, despite accurate histocompatibility typing and post-transplantation MTX. One patient developed GVH and recovered. Better techniques are obviously needed to select those patients who will develop a fatal GVH disease and better immunosuppressive regimens to prevent or treat it.

The CY regimen in these patients was well tolerated, except for Patient 8. Although the cause of his cardiac failure is not completely clear, the most likely explanation was CY toxicity, previously described in monkeys and man.[14,15]

These results should encourage earlier marrow grafting in patients with severe marrow failure who have HL-A matched siblings before major problems develop, with infection or hemorrhage, and before prior sensitization to transplantation antigens.

REFERENCES

1. Thomas, E. D., Lochte, H. L., Jr., Lu, W. C., and Ferrebee, J. W.: N. Engl. J. Med. 257:491, 1957.
2. Thomas, E. D., Rudolph, R. H., Fefer, A., Storb, R., Slichter, S., and Buckner, C. D.: Exp. Hematol. 21:16, 1971.
3. Thomas, E. D., Buckner, C. D., Storb, R., Neiman, P. E., Fefer, A., Clift, R. A., Slichter, S. J., Funk, D. D., Bryant, J. I., and Lerner, K. E.: Lancet 1:284, 1972.
4. Thomas, E. D., and Storb, R.: Blood 36:507, 1970.
5. Rudolph, R. H., Mickelson, E., and Thomas, E. D.: J. Clin. Invest. 49:2271, 1970.
6. Thomas, E. D., Buckner, C. D., Rudolph, R. H., Fefer, A., Storb, R., Neiman, P. E., Bryant, J. I., Chard, R. L., Clift, R. A., Epstein, R. B., Fialkow P. J., Funk, D. D., Giblett, E. R., Lerner, K. G., Reynolds, F. A., and Slichter, S.: Blood 38:267, 1971.
7. Fialkow, P. J., Thomas, E. D., Bryant, J. I., and Neiman, P. E.: Lancet 1:251, 1971.
8. Santos, G. W., Sensenbrenner, L. L., Burke, P. J., Colvin, M., Owens, A. H., Jr., Bias, W. B., and Slavin, R. E.: Transplant. Proc. 3:400, 1971.
9. Storb, R., Epstein, R. B., Graham, T. C., and Thomas, E. D.: Transplantation 9:240, 1970.
10. Buckner, C. D., Eisel, R., and Perry, S.: Blood 31:653, 1968.
11. Knospe, W. H., and Crosby, W. H.: Lancet 1:20, 1971.
12. Grumet, F. C., and Yankee, R. A.: Ann. Intern. Med. 73:1, 1970.
13. Storb, R., Rudolph, R. H., Graham, T. C., and Thomas, E. D.: J. Immunol. 107:409, 1971.
14. Storb, R., Buckner, C. D., Dillingham, L. A., and Thomas, E. D.: Cancer Res. 30:2195, 1970.
15. Buckner, C. D., Rudolph, R. H., Fefer, A., Clift, R. A., Epstein, R. B., Funk, D. D., Neiman, P. E., Slichter, S. J., Storb, R., and Thomas, E. D.: Cancer 29:357, 1972.

Marrow Grafting in Identical Twins With Hematologic Malignancies

A. Fefer, C. D. Buckner, R. A. Clift, L. Fass, K. G. Lerner,
E. M. Mickelson, P. Neiman, R. Rudolph, R. Storb, and E. D. Thomas

THE combination of lethal total body irradiation and normal syngeneic marrow has often been used to treat transplanted leukemias and lymphomas in mice, with only occasional effects in some animal models and no effect in most.[1] In man, acute leukemia is sometimes sensitive to total body irradiation and death from irradiation aplasia can be prevented by infusion of syngeneic marrow.[2] Therefore, in the late 1950's Thomas and collaborators[3,4] treated three patients with supralethal irradiation and normal syngeneic marrow. The results are shown in Table 1 above the horizontal line (nonnumbered patients). All three patients, all with acute lymphoblastic leukemia, exhibited recurrent leukemia within 48–84 days.

In an atempt to delay the rapid recurrence observed, various therapeutic modalities were added to the basic regimen of irradiation and marrow infusion. This report presents the results obtained by the Seattle Group during the past 3 years on a series of ten patients including five to be reported in detail elsewhere.[5] The results are summarized in Table 1. Each patient had a hematologic malignancy. Each was considered to have obtained maximum

Supported by Grant CA 10895, Training Grant CA 05231 and Contract PH 43-67-1435 from the USPHS, and by American Cancer Society Grant CI-52.

103

benefit from conventional chemotherapy and each had a normal twin whose identity was confirmed by dermatoglyphic studies, serotyping, blood genetic markers and mixed leukocyte culture tests. It must be emphasized that the changes in the therapeutic regimens evolved with time and the contribution of any given change to the end results observed could not be evaluated. The methodology involved, e.g. X-irradiation, marrow aspiration and transplantation, et cetera, has been previously described.[5]

One change involved additional chemotherapy. Patient 1 who was resistant to conventional chemotherapy, received 6 days of cytosine arabinoside therapy shortly before irradiation and marrow transplantation. On day 17 after the transplant, when his marrow was relatively hypoplastic but without evidence of leukemia, maintenance therapy with methotrexate (15 mg/sq m twice a week) was initiated. Unfortunately, leukemia still recurred on day 51.

Patient 2, whose diagnosis was somewhat in doubt but most likely was acute leukemia with some atypical features, received cyclophosphamide (CY) 60 mg/kg on each of 3 consecutive evenings, followed 5 days later by irradiation and marrow transplantation. A moderate decrease in skin nodules and in marrow involvement was observed within a week, but recurrence and progression was noted by day 16. Interestingly, despite the unusually vigorous combination of CY and irradiation, hemopoietic recovery (presumably engraftment) was rapid, with the peripheral white cell count rising to 1000/cu mm by day 12.

In a further effort to delay the recurrence of disease, potential immunotherapy was added to the treatment regimen of 8 patients. It was based rather loosely on

Table 1. Marrow Grafts in Identical Twins

Patient No.	Diagnosis	Age	Rx Before Grafting CY (mg/kg)	Irradiation (rad)	Immuno-therapy	Days to Recurrent Leukemia	Survival (Days)	Comments
1	ALL	4	—	748	—	84	450	These 3 patients were treated in 1958–1959[3,4]
	ALL	26	—	840	—	60	72	
	ALL	3	—	950	—	48	62	
	ALL	4	—	1000	—	51	85	Six days Rx with Ara-C before irradiation, MTX maintenance inltiated day 17
2	? Leukemia ? Undifferentiated tumor	37	180	1000	—	16	35	—
3	ALL	15	—	1000	+	33	97	Patient was one of a set of identical triplets
4	AML	33	—	1000	+	312	360	Died of interstitial pneumonitis. No evidence of leukemia at autopsy
5	AML	25	—	1000	+	—	51	—
6	Lymphosarcoma leukemia	19	120	1000	+	—	> 770	—
7	CML-Blast crisis	14	120	1000	+	104	> 297	Transplanted while in parital remission
8	ALL	13	120	1000	+	—	> 266	
9	AML	11	120	1000	+	—	> 239	Tumor cells injected 5 times, but no donor lymphocytes given
10	AML	18	120	1000	+	27	40	—

the assumed existence of tumor specific antigens on human leukemia cells, on studies in mice in which leukemia cells were eradicated by a combination of sublethal chemothrapy and syngeneic lymphocytes but only if the donors were immune to the antigens,[1] and on studies of active immunotherapy with leukemic cell vaccines in animals and man.[6] Accordingly, the recurrences observed after irradiation and syngeneic marrow infusion were interpreted as failures of immunotherapy due to the inability of nonimmune marrow to destroy residual leukemic cells, and one approach to potential immunotherapy was tried. It was based on several assumptions:

(1) Infusion of potentially immunologically reactive donor peripheral blood lymphocytes, presumably thymus-derived, might be beneficial.

(2) Lymphocytes immune to hypothetical leukemia antigens are preferable.

(3) Under the previous conditions either there were too few potentially reactive lymphocytes in the host to be immunized, or there was too little tumor to constitute an adequate immunogenic stimulus to the few cells, or the tumor cells in the host were not present in a form or extent or location for optimal immunogenicity.

(4) Administration of additional antigenic leukemia cells subcutaneously might be beneficial by immunizing donor lymphocytes in the host specifically or nonspecifically against leukemia antigens.

Accordingly, patients received irradiation and marrow and thereafter potential "immunotherapy" in the form of buffy coat lymphocytes from the identical twin about three times a week for about 3 wk plus weekly s.c. injections of their own leukemic cells stored at −180°C in 10% dimethyl sulfoxide and lethally X-irradiated with 10,000 rad. The results obtained in three patients (Cases, 3, 4, and 5) thus treated with irradiation, marrow transplantation, and immunotherapy are shown in Table 1. The immunotherapy consisted of a total of 32–39 billion lymphocytes and four to ten injections of tumor. Patient 3 rapidly exhibited recurrent leukemia, whereas Patient 4 experienced an 8-mo remission followed by recurrence. One patient with acute myelogenous leukemia had infectious problems before and after marrow transplantation, went into remission, but succumbed to an interstitial pneumonitis on day 51. At autopsy, no leukemia was evident.

It was assumed that the addition of a high dose of chemotherapy to the treatment regimen would be beneficial by decreasing the tumor load to be handled by irradiation and/or immunotherapy. Therefore, five patients (Cases 6–10) received CY 120 mg/kg before irradiation, marrow transplantation, and immunotherapy.

Patient 6 developed a lytic lesion of the hip in July 1969. On open biopsy it was diagnosed as lymphosarcoma. Marrow from the ilium and sternum revealed lymphoblastic infiltration indistinguishable from acute lymphoblastic leukemia. No lymphadenopathy or hepatosplenomegaly were noted. The patient was treated with chlorambucil, prednisone, and local irradiation with symptomatic relief. He then developed serious hypercalcemia and was treated with methotrexate, vincristine, and prednisone with complete remission, except that bone lesions failed to heal. In June 1970, he developed progressive pancytopenia with diffuse infiltration of the marrow with lymphoblasts, with hepatosplenomegaly and multiple osteolytic lesions and collapse of the fourth lumbar vertebra. His hematocrit was 32%, the white count 1900/cu mm and the platelet count

18,000/cu mm.

He received CY, 30 mg/kg, on each of 2 evenings and 60 mg/kg on the third. Five days later he received irradiation and twin marrow followed by 32×10^9 donor lymphocytes and ten weekly injections of irradiated tumor cells. The patient did very well, although his full hematologic recovery was slower than that of other patients. Twenty-six months after transplantation, he continued to attend college and is totally asymptomatic with normal hematologic counts and marrows and with no abnormal findings except that radiograms failed to show that lytic lesions were healing.

All subsequent patients received 60 mg/kg CY on each of two successive evenings. Two to 5 days later they received irradiation and marrow followed by immunotherapy. Patient 7, with chronic myelogenous leukemia in blast crisis, experienced only a brief remission when treated in this manner.

Patient 8 had been treated with numerous drug combinations with progressively shorter intervals to relapse. While in partial remission induced by L-asparaginase and cytosine arabinoside, she received CY, irradiation, and marrow, followed by seven units of donor lymphocytes—all in the first week—and 3 weekly injections of tumor cells. Her peripheral white count rose to 1000/cu mm by day 10' she went into complete remission, and remains so at 9 mo.

Patient 9 had acute promyelocytic leukemia unresponsive to a large variety of agents, developed leukemic skin nodules and presented rather ill with a hematocrit of 15%, a platelet count of 67,000, a white count of 1610/cu mm with a hypercellular marrow containing 90% blasts. He received the CY, irradiation, and marrow regimen as well as five injections of his own tumor cells. He did not, however, receive any identical twin lymphocytes because his twin had very poor veins. The patient exhibited a normal marrow by day 18 and remains in complete remission at 8 mo. By strong contrast, an 18-year-old man with acute myelogenous leukemia, unresponsive to a variety of agents, received the total regimen but did not respond, so that by day 26 his marrow contained 90% blasts.

Despite the small and rather heterogenous group of patients treated, several conclusions can be drawn from the results presented:

1. The entire procedure was remarkably well tolerated by the patients, with often no more toxicity than that observed with vigorous chemotherapy. Only one patient died without evidence of leukemia but with pneumonitis.

2. Engraftment was not a significant problem. All patients exhibited reasonable hemopoietic recovery, presumed though not proven to reflect engraftment of donor marrow and not simply recovery of host marrow.

3. The major problem was and is recurrent leukemia. Of the seven patients who died, six died with leukemia. It is assumed that the recurrences represented progeny of the original host leukemia cells. However the possibility of malignant transformation of infused donor cells, as documented in two leukemic recipients of alogeneic marrow grafts[7] cannot, of course, be ruled out.

4. The results do not permit one to attribute an effect or evaluate a contribution of a specific change in the treatment regimen to the total therapeutic results obtained. The immunotherapy, for example, may have contributed, greatly or alternatively, the additional lymphocytes,

killed tumor cells may have had no beneficial or a deleterious effect, and all results may simply reflect remission induction by more effective doses of irradiation and chemotherapy. Nevertheless, although the critical feature of the therapeutic regimen cannot be clearly pinpointed, the end-stage patients still alive and in unmaintained remission for 8, 9, and 26 mo, as well as the 8 mo long remission in another patient with acute myelogenous leukemia, are encouraging and gratifying and suggest that this approach or variation thereof has a place to the treatment of this unique group of patients with hematologic malignancies refractory to chemothrapy.

REFERENCES

1. Fefer, A.: Israel J. Med. Sci. (In press).
2. Thomas, E. D., Rudolph, R. H., Fefer, A., Storb, R., Slichter, S., and Buckner, C. D.: Exp. Hematol. 21:16, 1971.
3. Thomas, E. D., Herman, E. C., Jr., Greenough, W. B., III, Hager, E. B., Cannon, J. H., Sahler, O. D., and Ferrebee, J. W.: Arch. Int. Med. 107: 829, 1961.
4. Thomas, E. D., Lochte, H. L., Jr., Cannon, J. H., Sahler, O. D., and Ferrebee, J. W.: J. Clin. Invest. 38:1709, 1959.
5. Rudolph, R. H., Fefer, A., Thomas, E. D., Buckner, C. D., Clift, R. A., Epstein, R. B., Lutcher, C. L., Neiman, P., and Storb, R.: Arch. Int. Med. (In press).
6. Mathe, G.: Adv. Cancer Res. 14:1, 1971.
7. Storb, R., Bryant, J. I., Buckner, C. D., Clift, R. A., Fefer, A., Johnson, F. L., Neiman, P., and Thomas, E. D.: Transplant. Proc. this issue.

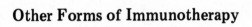

Other Forms of Immunotherapy

Transfer of Immune Responsiveness

W. H. Marshall, M.D., Ph.D.

The deliberate transfer of immune responsiveness is becoming commoner in medicine. There are three situations where transfers are used. Of particular interest are the *immunodeficiency diseases* where the aim of a transfer is to reconstitute the immune mechanism. Trials of transfer in these diseases are presently helping to throw light on the nature of the underlying deficiencies. In *infectious disease,* transfer has been used successfully to destroy an invading microorganism. Finally, the discovery that *tumors* may be antigenic to the host in which they are growing suggests that a powerful immune response against such antigens could be produced in the patient, perhaps by transfer, in order to eliminate the tumor.

There are alternative means of producing powerful immune responses that do not involve transfer of immunity; these are outside the scope of this paper. Such methods are direct immunization, the use of adjuvants, and the elimination of inhibitors of effective immune responses. Also outside its scope is a discussion of the transfer of immunity with serum antibody. The emphasis of this paper will be upon transfer of cells or cell extracts.

HISTORICAL DEVELOPMENT

Landsteiner and Chase in 1942[42] were the first to show that an immune response could be transferred with live lymphoid cells. They transferred contact sensitivity to simple chemicals in guinea pigs with viable lymphoid cells. The finding has since been confirmed in many species, including man, and with many different antigens.[14, 21]

The first demonstration of the transfer of transplantation immunity with lymphoid cells was made by Mitchison in 1954,[63] working with a transplantable tumor in mice. He coined the term "adoptive immunity" to describe this sort of transfer. In the same year, Harris et al.[36] reported the successful transfer, with lymphoid cells, of antibody-forming capability in rabbits.

113

When Lawrence began performing experimental transfers of delayed hypersensitivity in man, he discovered in 1954[13, 44] that, contrary to expectation, delayed hypersensitivity could be transferred by killed or even disrupted cells. This curious finding and the subsequent work of Lawrence and others on this "transfer factor" is summarized below, and has been reviewed in detail elsewhere by Lawrence.[45, 46, 49, 50]

PROBLEMS ARISING FROM CELL TRANSFER

There are two major problems that can be encountered if live lymphoid cells are transferred from one individual to another. The transferred cells, being immunologically competent, may mount an immune response against the host; alternatively, the grafted cells may be rejected by the host's own immune mechanism.

Graft-Versus-Host Disease

If the host's rejection mechanisms are absent, as for example in congenital T-cell deficiency, then the grafted lymphoid cells will survive and may themselves undertake a rejection reaction, rejecting the host in which they reside. This "graft-versus-host" (GVH) reaction is often fatal.

The fact that grafted lymphoid cells can actually attack the host in which they reside has been recognized in experimental animals for more than a decade. The extensive literature has been concisely summarized by Billingham.[13] The requirements for production of a graft-versus-host reaction are that graft and host differ antigenically, that the grafted lymphocytes are not destroyed in the host, and that a sufficiently large dose of cells is grafted. An important point, emerging from a study in rodents of the requirement for antigenic difference, is that there must be a major histocompatibility antigen involved, that is to say, an H-2 locus difference in mice or an Ag-B locus difference in rats. It is impossible to produce a lethal graft-versus-host reaction if one transfers cells between animals who share the same major antigens. The single exception to this statement is when the grafted cells are taken from an animal that has already been sensitized to host antigens; such "primed" cells can, and do, mount a graft-versus-host reaction against minor histocompatibility antigens.

Graft-versus-host reactions are now being recognized in human beings,[62] but, as will be evident later, man appears to be different from laboratory rodents. Bone marrow cells grafted between subjects who are apparently identical at the presumed major histocompatibility locus, HL-A, have unfortunately caused fatal graft-versus-host disease. The alternative interpretation of this conflict between findings in man and animals, although radical at this late stage, is that the main HL-A antigens in man have not yet been demonstrated; this challenging proposition has come from Snell, one of the most experienced workers in the field.[78]

Destruction of the Grafted Cells

If grafted cells contain an antigen which is foreign to the host into which they have been grafted, they will usually be destroyed by the host

114

immune response, a transplantation response. In the case of a free cell suspension, which in fact we are considering for the most part, there is the added hazard that serum antibody and complement may immediately destory the injected cells. Antibodies of this sort can easily be induced by prior transfusion or pregnancies.

Methods of Avoiding Unwanted Transplantation Reactions

The unwanted transplantation reactions—rejection of the graft and graft-versus-host disease—can be avoided in animal experiments by a number of strategies, and it is instructive to review some of them now so that the principles for solving similar problems in clinical situations become clear.

The transplantation response can be avoided completely, both for graft rejection and for graft-against-host reactions, if the animals are from the same inbred strain, that is to say, if there are no antigenic differences between the tissues of donor and recipient. In clinical practice as it stands today, a perfect match of this sort is found only between identical twins. However, the matching even of unrelated donor and recipient can, on rare occasions, be remarkably good.[29] Such matching is best achieved by a combination of serologic methods and the mixed leukocyte reaction.

Maneuvers that abolish the transplantation response can be listed in sequence according to the degree to which they achieve the specific result that is wanted. For example, whole-body X-irradiation and radiomimetic drugs are quite nonspecific. Corticosteroids spare many tissues but kill lymphocytes and depress inflammatory reactions. X-irradiation of the blood in an extracorporeal circuit,[20] on the other hand, will kill only blood cells and in so doing will sterilize the circulating lymphocytes. Cannulation of the thoracic duct with the formation of a chronic fistula is another way of getting rid of circulating lymphocytes;[54, 55] chronic local x-irradiation of the spleen does an even better job of destroying circulating lymphocytes.[31] Antilymphocyte serum destroys lymphocytes in both blood and tissues and, if the serum is monospecific, the other blood cells will be spared.[85] Finally, the induction of specific immunologic tolerance inactivates only those particular cells in the body which have the capability to respond to the antigen in question.

A completely different approach can be made with a specific "enhancing" antiserum.[11] Evidently, an appropriate serum against a transplantation antigen can hinder the access of lymphocytes to that antigen and thus prevent a transplantation response.

In experimental animals the above solutions can be used to overcome transplantation barriers, but in clinical medicine there are ethical problems as well since it is not easy to accept that a *donor* should be pretreated (although this has been done[59]) with drugs or antigen or x-irradiation, and so alternative methods have been sought. Cell separation by biophysical methods is presently being developed, the aim being to remove, from an inoculum, cells with unwanted activities. For example, potential graft-versus-host cells need to be removed if the inoculum is being injected into a patient with deficient cellular immunity.

It will be noted in the subsequent sections how much room there still is for improvements in cell transfer techniques simply by applying principles already well established in animal experimentation.

TRANSFER WITH SUBCELLULAR MATERIALS

Lawrence's transfer factor has the great advantage over inocula of live cells in that it will not produce graft-versus-host disease. However, the biological significance of transfer factor is still obscure and, as Burnet[19] recently wrote, the material poses "one of the outstanding conundrums of immunology." Since the original discovery that a state of sensitivity for delayed reactions could be transferred from one person to another with extracts of killed leukocytes, Lawrence has relentlessly repeated the experiment in a series of different systems, and has varied the experimental design in many ways, in order to meet the requests of his critics. However, because of the conceptual difficulties involved, it is likely that critics will remain until the chemical nature of transfer factor has been elucidated and its mechanism of action demonstrated.

Lawrence has performed transfers of sensitivity for a number of bacterial products, the prototype and the most easily transferred being tuberculin sensitivity; but, in spite of many years of careful work, the nature of the active material remains unknown. The reason for the delay is that there has been no laboratory animal in which transfer with disrupted cells can be achieved; in experiments in small laboratory mammals the cells must be alive for transfer to occur. Thus all analytical experiments have had to be made in human volunteers, and it is evident that if one uses tuberculin sensitivity, there will be rather few useful subjects (i.e., true tuberculin negative reactors) even in a large batch of volunteers. Whilst a biochemist might like to have a hundred tuberculin negative volunteers every week for assays, in practice it is usually possible to get negative subjects only in ones and twos.

So far as they have gone, experiments done to elucidate the chemical nature of transfer factor have simply added to the puzzle. For example, the material will pass through a dialysis membrane, which indicates that it has a molecular weight of less than 10,000, and in fact trials with chromatography suggest that it may be nearer to 5,000 M.W.[3, 9, 10, 47] This is very small for a specific "informational" molecule. Studies with enzymes have shown that transfer factor activity was not lost after incubation with either RNAse, DNAse, or trypsin. These treatments do not exclude the idea that transfer factor is low molecular weight double-stranded RNA; this appears to be the favorite hypothesis at present.

Lawrence has pursued the idea that transfer factor may be replicated within the body. In the first place, this could be suggested because the number of lysed leukocytes used for transfer is relatively small, the cells derived from 500 ml. of blood or less. This amount obviously represents only a tenth of the circulating blood and a very much smaller proportion of the total lymphoid tissue of the body, and yet this small amount of material converts the whole body of the recipient to a fair state of sensitivity. Lawrence has deliberately set out to find how long such a state of transferred sensitivity lasts, and in some cases of transfer of tuberculin sensitivity it lasted for the duration of the experiment, i.e., more than a year. This finding again points to the idea of self-replication. Finally, he has performed a few serial transfers to a third party and has been able to transfer tuberculin and streptococcal M substance sensitivities in this way.[45] Thus the concept of a small, highly specific, self-replicating molecule has gained ground. The only known molecules with the informational and replicating properties required are nucleic acids. In the case of transfer factor, the molecular weight is so small that only a few bases could be contained in each molecule, and that number would not be sufficient to dictate the required range of specificities, or any specificity for that matter if the conventional genetic code were employed for defining a conventional and complete antigen receptor site.

It is a curious finding that not all specificities are transferred with the same ease. There is in fact a rank order of antigens for the ease with which they are transferable. Tuberculin sensitivity is by far the easiest to transfer; in an intermediate category are diphtheria toxoid and streptococcal M substance sensitivity. Coccidioidin sensitivity is more difficult to transfer in spite of the fact that donors from endemic areas show very vigorous cutaneous reactions. In his study of transfer of coccidioidin sensitivity,[72] Lawrence only obtained regular success in transfer when he mixed equal quantities of positive transfer factor with coccidioidin itself. Such a maneuver looks suspiciously like immunization; however, Lawrence obtained evidence that the transfer factor did play a specific role, since, when he used truly negative transfer factor, there was no sensitization with a coccidioidin-transfer factor mixture. Homograft sensitivity similarly presented problems when Lawrence tried transfers after sensitizing a leukocyte donor with a skin graft.[48] He eventually found it was possible to transfer homograft sensitivity only by taking leukocytes from the donor during the process of rejection of the fourth of a series of skin grafts. Finally, when we come to consider contact chemical sensitivity in which prior skin testing of the recipient is excluded and which is a classic sensitivity transferable by cells in the guinea pig, it must be admitted that a serious attempt by Brandriss[16] to transfer this sensitivity in man, with dialysed transfer factor, showed absolutely no transfer. This result was despite successful concurrent transfer of tuberculin sensitivity to the test subjects with the same transfer factor preparation. Whether this represents a more "difficult" sensitivity to transfer or whether there is a qualitative difference is unknown; it is possible that, since the sensitivity is to a chemical sensitizer bound to tissue, there may be important antigenic differences between the tissue of the donor in whom the sensitivity was clearly demonstrable and the recipient who failed to show sensitivity. It is known that the "carrier" of a hapten has to be identical to that used for immunization for there to be demonstrable delayed hypersensitivity to a hapten-protein conjugate on cutaneous testing.

The present attack on the transfer factor problem is being carried on *in vitro*. For example, Baram and Condoulis[8] have been able to induce nonsensitized cells to behave as if they had been sensitized, by culturing them together with a lysate of sensitive cells; so far, though, they have had no positive results using the small molecular weight material prepared by dialysis. In Lawrence's laboratory, Valentine[82] had negative or minimally positive results in attempts to alter the reactivity of cultured lymphocytes by adding dialysable transfer factor, but he has now discovered that sensitive cells can release a material into the culture medium which in its action is tantalizingly like transfer factor. The experiment involves culturing sensitive leukocytes with antigen and then taking the culture medium and placing it in a fresh culture tube together with some lymphocytes which are known to be not sensitive to the antigen in question. These nonsensitive leukocytes are now found to respond to the antigen by growing into lymphoblasts which divide. Valentine has done the experiment in various ways to show that the response is both antigen dependent and antigen specific. Further analyses of this experiment are awaited with interest.

There is a whole branch of scientific literature devoted to the laboratory artifact of adding nucleic acids to cells of a certain genetic constitution and watching them perform differently under the influence of the added genetic information. Experiments of this sort involving immune systems have been reviewed in a symposium,[71] and it suffices to describe one recent experiment to indicate what can happen. Bell and Dray[12] took normal spleen cells from a rabbit and incubated them in the presence of RNA extracted from another rabbit spleen at the height of an immune response against sheep red blood cells. Presumably some of the RNA entered these normal spleen cells because a large number of antibody-forming cells appeared which were making antibody against sheep red cells. That the antibody synthesis had been directed by the donor RNA was neatly demonstrated by showing that the antibody was of the allotype appropriate to the donor spleen rather than to the normal spleen cells. Whether the donated RNA becomes transmitted to subsequent generations of cells is an open question, but the existence in transformed lymphocytes of an enzyme capable of making new DNA from an RNA template[70] would allow such a genetic transformation to occur.

It is sometimes argued that both the transfer factor experiments and the *in vitro* experiments with RNA are artifacts of the experimentalist and bear no relationship to biological reality. That may be, but from a therapeutic point of view a successfully transferred response is what is aimed at, no matter if it is an artificial or unnatural maneuver.

TREATMENT OF CONGENITAL IMMUNODEFICIENCY BY TRANSFER

If one excludes from this discussion defects of nonspecific immunity (e.g., complement or phagocytosis defects), one is left with congenital defects in specific immunity, of which there are three main groups: (1) agammaglobulinemia, (2) absence of specific cell-mediated immunity typified by the DiGeorge syndrome, and (3) combined deficiency where there is a lack both of immunoglobulins and of specific cell-mediated immunity. Agammaglobulinemia has been reasonably effectively treated with replacement injections of immunoglobulin,[51, 60] and there has been little justification for trials of cell transfer; this group of diseases will therefore receive no further mention, except to note that in one revealing case, a patient was treated with bone marrow transfusions from an identical twin, with no lasting restoration.[23] The treatment of the latter two syndromes has been primarily by transfer of immune responsiveness, and it is pertinent to review what has been achieved. At the end of this section the Wiskott-Aldrich syndrome will also be considered.

DiGeorge Syndrome

Attempts to treat the DiGeorge syndrome are recent and make an exciting story. In 1968, two cases were treated, both in the United States.

The Miami case[22] involved an infant who had had recurrent infections and diarrhea as well as a troublesome hypocalcemia. No thymic shadow was demonstrable even by pneumomediastinography. A fetal thymus was transplanted into the rectus abdominis muscle. By the next day the lymphocyte count had risen from 1300 to 5600. Subsequently it was found that dinitro-chlorobenzene (DNCB) sensitivity appeared spontaneously (earlier attempts at sensitization had failed) and "within a few weeks after the transplant, diarrhoea and rhinorrhoea ceased." The boy was observed for 18 months and remained restored and well.

The Boston case[5] was a typical case of DiGeorge syndrome with absence of thymus on x-ray, right-sided aortic arch. and other anomalies. In this patient, as in the Miami case, DNCB sensitivity and other delayed sensitivities appeared spontaneously after transplantation of a thymus from a 16-week fetus. The lymphocyte responses to phytohemagglutinin (PHA) were studied extensively; there was a minimal response before transplantation, which was restored to normal 4 days after transplantation. Of great interest was the finding, by use of the sex chromosome marker, that the cells responding to PHA were the patient's own; in some fashion, possibly hormonal, the thymus transplant had endowed his own lymphocytes with the ability to respond to PHA. This patient, too, has been followed for over a year and remains well and fully restored.[4]

Combined Immunodeficiency

Treatment of this malignant condition has proved to be difficult, and it is interesting to review chronologically the published attempts, since they show the way in which ideas have developed.

A patient was treated in Boston by thymic transplant as early as 1962,[74] only a year after the first description of the effect of neonatal thymectomy in mice. A piece of thymus from a 5 month old child, obtained during a heart operation, was transplanted but without any effect. In 1965 Swiss workers[37] treated two patients by transplantation of fetal thymus. The results in one patient showed that such a transplant could survive, since healthy thymus was later found at necropsy after two thymuses and some fetal bone marrow cells had been administered without effect. The second patient had a total of 11 fetal thymuses transplanted and on one occasion some fetal liver cells. The fetal liver injection was followed by restoration of the blood lymphocyte count, but DNCB sensitization was not possible, the cells failed to respond in culture to PHA, and the patient died at 6 months of age.

In 1966 a group in Oslo[35] transplanted a thymus from a 16 week old fetus. A monoclonal gammopathy developed in the patient subsequently, and this protein was thought, from Gm typing, to have originated from cells of the donor and not of the patient. However, the patient became ill with an erythematous rash and died. The French experience with thymus transplantation in one case was equally disappointing.[56]

In 1966 and 1967, 2 patients in the United States were given injections of maternal bone marrow cells. One child[62] developed a fulminant graft-against-host syndrome (which was beginning to be recognized by this time) and died. The other child's[75] lymphocyte count rose 1 week after transplantation, with more than half of the cells being of infant origin as shown by sex chromosome analysis. Furthermore, the child developed a cutaneous sensitivity to Monilia antigen. However, the patient died some 13 days after transplantation, from multiple causes, including infection.

In 1968 a similar case was reported from Minnesota.[39] The infant was given fetal thymus and liver cells plus a transfusion of fresh maternal blood. Within days there was evidence of immunologic restoration, but this was shortly followed by a recognizable graft-versus-host syndrome, and the patient died.

It was evident from these cases of graft-versus-host disease that better histocompatibility matching would be needed, and it was hoped that a complete match at the main locus (HL-A) would be sufficient[38] (see above). HL-A-compatible siblings were considered to be the most promising sources of compatible bone marrow.

In 1969, after 7 years of failures, there were at last sporadic successes. A patient was treated in Minnesota[61] by sibling bone marrow and was apparently restored by a second marrow transplant after the first had induced a state of aplastic anemia. A patient was treated in Holland[26] with HL-A-compatible sibling bone marrow; however, the Dutch workers introduced a further modification in the procedure, namely, the "purification" of the bone marrow cell suspension on a density gradient to remove the majority of graft-versus-host cells. The patient had a mild graft-versus-host reaction with a morbilliform rash but ultimately did well. Two further patients have been treated; in one[11] a bone marrow transplant from a sibling caused a fatal graft-versus-host reaction; the other was treated by The Ontario Cancer Institute group,[1] who attempted to remove graft-versus-host cells by a cell separation method involving differential sedimentation. While there was no restoration of the defect in the Canadian patient, there was no graft-versus-host disease either.

An atypical case of combined deficiency was recently managed[2] successfully with two marrow transplants from an HL-A identical sibling. A delayed graft-versus-host reaction resolved spontaneously, and the child has done well for a year.

The occurrence of graft-versus-host reaction, even with bone marrow grafts from HL-A compatible siblings, encouraged further trials of fetal liver cells but these have met with no success.[33, 34]

Another interesting approach is mentioned in a recent World Health Organization report;[51] in 2 patients an enhancing antiserum was injected into the bone marrow recipient in order to prevent the grafted cells from mounting a graft-versus-host response, the idea being that the antibody conceals the host's transplantation antigens.

120

Thus, at the time of writing, despite many years of unfruitful experiment, the outlook is now good. Several patients have evidently been cured with bone marrow transplants, and we can expect that further technical refinements will soon allow many more persons to be cured.

The Wiskott-Aldrich Syndrome

This syndrome is characterized by eczema, thrombocytopenia, and recurrent infections. Both bone marrow transplantation and injections of Lawrence's transfer factor have been tried in order to correct this condition. Bach et al.[7] gave HL-A compatible marrow from a sibling and apparently effected both a cure and the establishment of a chimeric state as regards the blood cells. The patient's eczema cleared, infections regressed, and the platelet count rose from about 7500 per cu. mm. to around 17,500, and he has apparently remained well for nearly 2 years.[6]

An interesting approach was that of Levin and Spitler and their colleagues,[52, 53, 79] who prepared transfer factor from healthy individuals and injected it into patients with this syndrome. In 3 out of 5 cases there was marked improvement in the clinical state although the platelet counts were not dramatically altered. In the remaining 2 patients there was no response. Further trials of this safe and simple form of treatment are awaited with interest.

TREATMENT OF INFECTIOUS DISEASE BY TRANSFER

When an infection overwhelms an individual there is, almost by definition, an immunologic deficit in the sense that the immune response is inadequate to the task of destroying the infectious agent. Thus the consideration of infections as separate from immune deficiency states is somewhat artificial; however, there are several well documented instances where transfer of immunity has been used in the treatment of specific infections, so that is is convenient to consider these separately. It is probable that the use of cell transfer to overcome troublesome infections is commoner than the literature would suggest, since many instances of leukocyte transfusions may go unreported. For example, an overwhelming infection with varicella virus in a patient with leukemia or lymphoma can sometimes be cured by giving the patient a transfusion of blood leukocytes or bone marrow from a healthly individual – preferably, of course, one who has recently emerged from the convalescent period after an attack of chicken pox.

Generalized Vaccinia

Kempe[40] has reported a dramatic case in which generalized vaccinia occurred in a child following smallpox vaccination and progressed to the lethal stage termed vaccinia necrosum. There was no improvement after huge doses of hyperimmune globulin, and the child's arm eventually needed amputation. The generalized infection continued unabated until buffy coat leukocytes from three recently vaccinated adult donors were injected locally round the amputation site and the cells from three lymph nodes from similar donors were given intravenously and a further three lymph nodes were implanted in the rectus abdominis muscle. Kempe amply documents the regression of the infection and reports that there was no recurrence during the succeeding year.

O'Connell et al.[67] treated an elderly lady with progressive vaccinia which involved skin and mucous membranes. After other measures, including immune globulin, had failed, they gave her an injection of washed leukocytes from 250 ml. of blood obtained from a recently vaccinated donor. This transfer was apparently responsible for regression of the lesions and return of the patient to good health. A recurrence of one lesion on the foot occurred a month later, and was treated with a second injection of washed leukocytes with the same gratifying result—a huge ulcer healed almost completely in a matter of 2 weeks.

Chronic Mucocutaneous Candidiasis

This condition may be found in clearly defined immunodeficiency states such as the DiGeorge syndrome, but in many cases the nature of the underlying defect is obscure and there may be a group of different defects. The treatment for the most part remains empirical and experimental. Some success with cell transfer has been described, and attempts have been made to treat this condition with leukocyte extracts.

Buckley et al.[17] treated a 10 year old patient who had had the condition all her life. All other treatments having failed, they gave her a transfusion of bone marrow cells from her father. The result was impressive, with clearance of the candida infection and a growth spurt raising her from the third percentile to between the tenth and twenty-fifth percentiles, and she remained well for over a year.

Attempts have been made to use transfer factor, but the clinical results have been mixed. Rocklin et al.[73] gave dialysable transfer factor and showed that there was a temporary conversion of the delayed skin reaction to candida, and the patient's lymphocytes responded to the antigen in vitro by producing migration inhibition factor (MIF) but the infection did not improve. Another patient[37] was given dialysable transfer factor from very sensitive donors on 5 separate occasions, but there was no clinical improvement and no conversion of his negative skin test even after a final injection of whole leukocyte lysate. Spitler et al.,[80] on the other hand, have treated 3 patients and found clinical improvement in all of them, although extensive testing of lymphocytes before and after transfer failed to show any consistent defects or changes resulting from treatment. Similarly Schulkind et al.[77] found transfer factor to be beneficial in their patient.

Leprosy

The prognosis of leprosy is considerably better when the patient shows delayed hypersensitivity to lepromin than when such hypersensitivity is absent. It was therefore suggested[28] that transfer of immunity might be good treatment. De Bonaparte et al.[25] were able to convert 5 of 13 lepromatous patients to a sensitive state by transfer of leukocytes from positive reactors. Similarly transfer has been achieved with transfer factor.[18] In neither case is it yet possible to state whether the clinical course of the patients was significantly improved.

TREATMENT OF TUMORS BY TRANSFER

Immunotherapy of cancer, which includes the transfer of immune responsiveness as one of its techniques, acquired a sound theoretical basis once it was recognized that tumors may contain antigens not present in the host and that there may be evidence of an immune response in the host directed against the tumor. It was realized that this response could, potentially at any rate, destroy the tumor.

Methods of immunotherapy other than by transfer have been reviewed elsewhere.[30, 59, 64, 68]

The use of transfer in the treatment of human cancer is in an early stage, but there is every reason to believe that the initial approach can be refined. In general, there have been two approaches: (1) transfer normal lymphoid cells (or cell products) in the hope that these might mount an attack on the tumor; (2) remove tumor cells and use them to immunize either an animal or another human in order to obtain "immune" lymphoid cells which can then be transferred to the patient.

Transfer of Normal Cells

The pioneers of this method were Woodruff and Nolan,[86] who injected large numbers of normal spleen cells into patients with advanced or terminal cancer. The spleens were obtained from the operating room, having been removed for a variety of reasons, and were reduced to cell suspensions for intravenous or intraperitoneal injection. Despite the advanced stage of disease and despite the fact that there was no prior exposure of the spleen cells to tumor antigens, there was in every case some evidence suggestive of a temporary attack on the tumor. For example, cutaneous metastases became inflamed and partly necrotic, and in the case of peritoneal metastases there was a temporary regression in the rate of ascites formation. The authors suggested that the grafted cells had become sensitized to the tumor and had produced a destructive "graft-against-tumor" response.

Other workers have continued these experiments,[81] with the modification that they used spleen cells which had been stored frozen. Their results were essentially similar to the earlier work, but the authors were more impressed with results obtained using immunized pig lymphocytes (see below).

Mathé and his group[59] have tried inducing graft-against-tumor effects in the treatment of acute leukemia. They took 21 patients and gave them transfusions of large numbers of leukocytes from patients with chronic myeloid leukemia. They report obtaining remissions in 9 of the patients and, in 5, these were described as "complete." Subsequent attempts to produce the same remissions using vast numbers of lymphocytes from healthy volunteers were disappointing. The authors suggested that there was something particularly beneficial in the use of chronic myeloid leukemia cells for such transfusions.

Immunization of the Leukocyte Donor

USING HUMAN BEINGS. Nadler and Moore[66] took pairs of patients with malignant tumors and immunized each member with a piece of the other's tumor. After about 5 days, leukocyte transfers were begun. The cells from 500 ml. blood of each member of the pair were removed and were injected into the other member of the pair, and this process was repeated daily for 3 weeks. In their series of 85 patients, 53 were considered suitable for inclusion in the final analysis of results. Of these 13 had clear objective evidence of improvement and two remarkable patients were apparently cleared completely of their disease.

Other groups are preparing to perform similar trials; for example, a group in Texas[24] has completed preliminary baseline experiments to establish satisfactory transfer routines.

USING ANIMALS. Symes et al.[81] immunized pigs with tumor biopsy material and then, at the height of a presumed immune response, removed all the draining lymph nodes and made from them a lymphocyte suspension. The cells were then injected into the patient. In the 2 patients who received this therapy, there was apparently a striking improvement which lasted 4 to 6 weeks, but ultimately both patients died of their disease.

Use of Subcellular Materials

Two trials have recently been made in the use of transfer factor for tumor immunotherapy. Brandes et al.[15] used the cross-immunization design of Nadler and Moore in 2 patients with advanced malignant melanoma, and transfer factor was exchanged between members of the pair. Significant but temporary improvement was reported. A group in New York[69] have used transfer factor from healthy middle-aged women to treat breast cancer, arguing that breast cancers are likely to arise in many women and be eliminated by an immune response in most of them. Thus anti-tumor activity could be predicted to occur in such transfer factor preparations. In 1 of their 5 patients, the progress of the disease was halted for 6 months.

POSSIBLE FUTURE TRENDS

Removal of Cells of Certain Specificities

Cell separation by biophysical methods exploits differences in cell size and cell density, but neither of these is in any sense immunologically specific. There are, however, ways of separating cells on the basis of immunologic specificity; for example, Wigzell[84] has devised *antigen-loaded columns*. He attaches an antigen to a filter material in a column and then runs a cell suspension slowly through the column and finds that cells with specific receptors for the antigen adhere to the column and can be removed from the rest of the suspension. Hopefully transplantation antigens will one day be used in this way to remove cells with a certain transplantation response capability.

Another way to remove specific cells is to use the *"hot pulse" method* devised by Dutton.[27] Here the object is to stimulate a cell suspension with an antigen and then, when specifically reactive cells have responded by starting to divide, a large dose of tritiated thymidine is added to the culture. The dividing cells will then take up a disabling or even lethal dose of radioactivity. In fact, a first attempt to use this method in a clinical situation has been briefly reported.[76] One can visualize other modifications of this general approach, for example, the large dividing cells might be separated from the rest of the suspension by a biophysical method; this, indeed, has already been done in mice by Dutton.[27]

Enriching for a Certain Specificity

In the treatment of infectious disease or tumors, one needs a large number of cells possessing one particular specificity. Since it is known that antigen-stimulated cells can form quite large clones *in vitro* by repeated division,[58] it may be possible by careful tissue culture to grow vast numbers of cells with the single required specificity and then return them to the patient. Certainly the technology has now been developed for growing phenomenal numbers of cells in culture,[65] and indeed cultured leukocytes have been found to produce an occasional cell line which divides continuously. The specific reactivity, if any, of these lines is unknown, but attempts have been made to stimulate such a line with tumor antigen before returning the cells to the patient.[65] The ineffectiveness of this treatment was presumably because the tumor antigens failed, at that late stage, to direct the immunologic activity of the cell line.

SUMMARY

It is possible to transfer immune responsiveness with cells of the lymphatic system and, in certain cases, with RNA or other material extracted from the lymphoid cells (Lawrence's transfer factor). The hazard of graft-versus-host disease is avoided if cell extracts are used, but the potency of extracts may be less than that of live cells in some cases.

In *immunodeficiency disease*, (1) thymus transplantation has been used successfully to reconstitute two patients with the DiGeorge syndrome, (2) recent developments in bone marrow transplantation are improving the outlook for treatment of the combined immunodeficiency syndrome, and (3) the Wiskott-Aldrich syndrome has been ameliorated with bone marrow cells and with transfer factor. In *infectious disease*, transfer of immunity has been valuable in progressive vaccinia, in some cases of mucocutaneous candidiasis, and it has been possible to convert lepromin negative lepers to a lepromin positive state. *Cancer immunotherapy* by cell transfer is in its early stages, but even so the results are encouraging, and there have been two cases where complete disappearance of malignant melanoma was associated with cell transfer.

Future trends will involve treatment of inocula of cells to remove cells with unwanted specificities and to enrich for cells of the required specificity.

REFERENCES

1. Amato, D., Bergsagel, D. E., Clarysse, A. M., Cowan, D. H., Iscove, N. N., McCulloch, E. A., Miller, R. G., Phillips, R. A., Ragab, A. H., and Senn, J. S.: Review of bone marrow transplants at the Ontario Cancer Institute. Transplant. Proc., 3:397–399, 1971.
2. Ammann, A. J., Meuwissen, H. J., Good, R. A., and Hong, R.: Successful bone marrow transplantation in a patient with humoral and cellular immunity deficiency. Clin. Exper. Immunol., 7:343–353, 1970.

3. Arala-Chaves, M. P., Lebacq, E. G., and Heremans, J. F.: Fraction of human leukocyte extracts transferring delayed hypersensitivity to tuberculin. Int. Arch. Allergy, 31:353-365, 1967.
4. August, C. S., Berkel, A. I., Levey, R. H., Rosen, F. S., and Kay, H. E. M.: Establishment of immunological competence in a child with congenital thymic aplasia by a graft of fetal thymus. Lancet, 1:1080-1083, 1970.
5. August, C. S., Rosen, F. S., Filler, R. M., Janeway, C. A., Markowski, B., and Kay, H. E. M.: Implantation of a foetal thymus, restoring immunological competence in a patient with thymic aplasia. Lancet, 2:1210-1211, 1968.
6. Bach, F. H.: Personal communication, cited by Levin et al.[52]
7. Bach, F. H., Albertini, R. J., Anderson, J. L., Joo, P., and Bortin, M. M.: Bone-marrow transplantation in a patient with the Wiskott-Aldrich syndrome. Lancet, 2:1364-1366, 1968.
8. Baram, P., and Condoulis, W.: Transfer of delayed hypersensitivity to rhesus monkey and human lymphocytes with transfer factor obtained from rhesus monkey peripheral white blood cells. J. Immunol., 104:769-779, 1970.
9. Baram, P., and Mosko, M. M.: A dialysable fraction from tuberculin-sensitive human white blood cells capable of inducing tuberculin-delayed sensitivity in negative recipients. Immunology, 8:461-474, 1965.
10. Baram, P., Yuan, L., and Mosko, M. M.: Studies on the transfer of human delayed-type hypersensitivity. I. Partial purification and characterization of two active components. J. Immunol., 97:407-420, 1966.
11. Batchelor, J. R., Ellis, F., French, M. E., Bewick, M., Cameron, J. S., and Ogg, C. S.: Immunological enhancement of human kidney graft. Lancet, 2:1007-1010, 1970.
12. Bell, C., and Dray, S.: Conversion of non-immune spleen cells by ribonucleic acid of lymphoid cells from an immunized rabbit to produce γy-M antibody of foreign light chain allotype. J. Immunol., 103:1196-1211, 1969.
13. Billingham, R. E.: The biology of graft-versus-host reactions. In Harvey Lectures, Series 62, 1966-1967. New York, Academic Press, 1968, pp. 21-78.
14. Bloom, B. R., and Chase, M. W.: Transfer of delayed-type hypersensitivity: A critical review and experimental study in the guinea pig. In Kallós, P., and Waksman, B. H., eds.: Progress in Allergy. Basel and New York, S. Karger, 1967, vol. X, pp. 151-255.
15. Brandes, L. J., Galton, D. A. G., and Wiltshaw, E.: New approach to immunotherapy of melanoma. Lancet, 2:293-295, 1971.
16. Brandriss, M. W.: Attempt to transfer contact hypersensitivity in man with dialysate of peripheral leukocytes. J. Clin. Invest., 47:2152-2157, 1968.
17. Buckley, R. H., Lucas, Z. J., Hattler, B. G., Jr., Zmijewski, C. M., and Amos, D. B.: Defective cellular immunity associated with chronic mucocutaneous moniliasis and recurrent staphylococcal botryomycosis: Immunological reconstitution by allogeneic bone marrow. Clin. Exper. Immunol., 3:153-169, 1968.
18. Bullock, W. E., Fields, J., and Brandriss, M.: Transfer factor therapy in lepromatous leprosy: An evaluation. J. Clin. Invest., 50:16a, 1971.
19. Burnet, M.: In Cellular Immunology. Carlton, Australia, and Great Britain, Melbourne University Press and Cambridge University Press, 1969, book 1, p. 254.
20. Chanana, A. D., Brecher, G., Cronkite, E. P., Joel, D., and Schnappauf, H.: The influence of extracorporeal irradiation of the blood and lymph on skin homograft rejection. Radiat. Res., 27:330-346, 1966.
21. Chase, M. W.: Delayed sensitivity. MED. CLIN. N. AMER., 49:1613-1646, 1965.
22. Cleveland, W. W., Fogel, B. J., Brown, W. T., and Kay, H. E. M.: Foetal thymic transplant in a case of DiGeorge's syndrome. Lancet, 2:1211-1214, 1968.
23. Cruchaud, A., Girard, J.-P., Kapanci, Y., Laperrouza, C., Mégevand, R., and Schwarzenberg, L.: Agammaglobulinémie chez un seul de deux jumeaux univitellins: Description et tentatives thérapeutiques par transfusion de cellules immunocompétentes isologues. Rev. Franç. Clin. Biol., 13:245-257, 1968.
24. Curtis, J. E., Hersh, E. M., and Freireich, E. J.: Antigen-specific immunity in recipients of leukocyte transfusions from immune donors. Cancer Res., 30:2921-2929, 1970.
25. DeBonaparte, Y., Morgenfeld, M. C., and Paradisi, E. R.: Immunology of leprosy. New Eng. J. Med., 279:49, 1968.
26. DeKoning, J., van Bekkum, B. W., Dicke, K. A., Dooren, L. J., van Rood. J. J., and Rádl, J.: Transplantation of bone-marrow cells and fetal thymus in an infant with lymphopenic immunological deficiency. Lancet, 1:1223-1227, 1969.
27. Dutton, R. W., and Mishell, R. I.: Cellular events in the immune response. The in vitro response of normal spleen cells to erythrocyte antigens. Cold Spring Harbor Symposium Quant. Biol., 32:407-414, 1967.
28. Editorial: Transfer factor and leprosy. New Eng. J. Med., 278:333, 1968.
29. Eijsvoogel, V. P., Schellekens, P. T. A., Breur-Vriesendorp, B., Koning, L., Koch, C., van Leeuwen, A., and van Rood, J. J.: Mixed lymphocyte cultures and HL-A. Transplant. Proc., 3:85-88, 1971.
30. Fairley, G. H.: Immunity to malignant disease in man. In The Scientific Basis of Medicine Annual Reviews. London, Athlone Press, 1971, pp. 17-38.

31. Ford, W. L.: The mechanism of lymphopenia produced by chronic irradiation of the rat spleen. Brit. J. Exper. Path., 49:502–510, 1968.
32. Gatti, R. A., Meuwissen, H. J., Allen, H. D., Hong, R., and Good, R. A.: Immunological reconstitution of sex-linked lymphopenic immunological deficiency. Lancet, 2:1366–1369, 1968.
33. Gatti, R. A., Platt, N., Pomerance, H. H., Hong, R., Langer, L. O., Kay, H. E. M., and Good, R. A.: Hereditary lymphopenic agammaglobulinemia associated with a distinctive form of short-limbed dwarfism and ectodermal dysplasia. J. Pediat., 75:675–684, 1969.
34 Githens, J. H., Muschenheim, F., Fulginiti, V. A., Robinson, A., and Kay, H. E. M.: Thymic alymphoplasia with XX/XY lymphoid chimerism secondary to probable maternal-fetal transfusion. J. Pediat., 75:87–94, 1969.
35. Harboe, M., Pande, H., Brandtzaeg, P., Tveter, K. J., and Hjort, P. F.: Synthesis of donor type G-globulin following thymus transplantation in hypo-globulinaemia with severe lymphocytopenia. Scand. J. Haemat., 3:351–374, 1966.
36. Harris, S., Harris, T. N., and Farber, M. B.: Studies on the transfer of lymph node cells. I. Appearance of antibody in recipients of cells from donor rabbits injected with antigen. J. Immunol., 72:148–160, 1954.
37. Hitzig, W. H., Kay, H. E. M., and Cottier, H.: Familial lymphopenia with agammaglobulinaemia: An attempt at treatment by implantation of foetal thymus. Lancet, 2:151–154, 1965.
38. Hong, R., Gatti, R. A., and Good, R. A.: Hazards and potential benefits of blood-transfusion in immunological deficiency. Lancet, 2:388–389, 1968.
39. Hong, R., Kay, H. E. M., Cooper, M. D., Meuwissen, H., Allan, M. J. G., and Good, R. A.: Immunological restitution in lymphopenic immunological deficiency syndrome. Lancet, 1:503–506, 1968.
40. Kempe, C. H.: Studies on smallpox and complications of smallpox vaccination. Pediatrics, 26:176–189, 1960.
41. Kretschmer, R., Jeannet, M., Mereu, T. R., Kretschmer, K., Winn, H., and Rosen, F. S.: Hereditary thymic dysplasia: A graft-versus-host reaction induced by bone marrow cells with a partial 4a series histoincompatibility. Pediat. Res., 3:34–40, 1969.
42. Landsteiner, K., and Chase, M. W.: Experiments on transfer of cutaneous sensitivity to simple chemical compounds. Proc. Soc. Exper. Biol., New York, 49:688–690, 1942.
43. Lawrence, H. S.: The transfer of generalized cutaneous hypersensitivity of the delayed tuberculin type in man by means of the constituents of disrupted leucocytes. J. Clin. Invest., 33:951–952, 1954.
44. Lawrence, H. S.: The transfer in humans of delayed skin sensitivity to streptococcal M substance and to tuberculin with disrupted leucocytes. J. Clin. Invest., 34:219–230, 1955.
45. Lawrence, H. S.: Transfer factor. Adv. Immunol., 11:195–266, 1969.
46. Lawrence, H. S.: Transfer factor and cellular immune deficiency disease. New Eng. J. Med., 283:411–419, 1970.
47. Lawrence, H. S., Al-Askari, S., David, J., Franklin, E. C., and Zweiman, B.: Transfer of immunological information in humans with dialysates of leucocyte extracts. Trans. Assoc. Amer. Phys., 76:84–91, 1963.
48. Lawrence, H. S., Rapaport, F. T., Converse, J. M., and Tillett, W. S.: Transfer of delayed hypersensitivity to skin homografts with leukocyte extracts in man. J. Clin. Invest., 39:185–198, 1960.
49. Lawrence, H. S., and Valentine, F. T.: Transfer factor and other mediators of cellular immunity. Amer. J. Path., 60:437–451, 1970.
50. Lawrence, H. S., and Valentine, F. T.: Transfer factor in delayed hypersensitivity. Ann. N.Y. Acad. Sci., 169:269–280, 1970.
51. Leading Article: Variable immunodeficiency. Lancet, 1:959–960, 1971.
52. Levin, A. S., Spitler, L. E., Stites, D. P., and Fudenberg, H. H.: Wiskott-Aldrich syndrome, a genetically determined cellular immunologic deficiency: Clinical and laboratory responses to therapy with transfer factor. Proc. Nat. Acad. Sci., 67:821–828, 1970.
53. Levin, A. S., Spitler, L. E., Stites, D. P., and Fudenberg, H. H.: Molecular intervention in genetically determined cellular immune deficiency disorders. J. Clin. Invest., 50:59a, Abstr. 196, 1971.
54. McGregor, D. D., and Gowans, J. L.: The antibody response of rats depleted of lymphocytes by chronic drainage from the thoracic duct. J. Exper. Med., 117:303–320, 1963.
55. McGregor, D. D., and Gowans, J. L.: Survival of homografts of skin in rats depleted of lymphocytes by chronic drainage from the thoracic duct. Lancet, 1:629–632, 1964.
56. Marie, J., Hennequet, A., Jarlier, H., Cloup, M., Watchi, J.-M., and Allaneau, C.: Alymphocytose congénitale. Greffe thymique de 28°. Jour. Ann. Pediat., Paris, 13:804–811, 1968.
57. Marshall, W. H., and Darte, J. M. M.: Unpublished observations, 1971.
58. Marshall, W. H., Valentine, F. T., and Lawrence, H. S.: Cellular immunity in vitro. J. Exper. Med., 130:327–343, 1969.
59. Mathé, G.: Approaches to the immunological treatment of cancer in man. Brit. Med. J., 4:7–10, 1969.

127

60. Medical Research Council Special Report Series No. 310: Hypogammaglobulinaemia in the United Kingdom. London, Her Majesty's Stationery Office, 1971.
61. Meuwissen, H. J., Gatti, R. A., Terasaki, P. I., Hong, R., and Good, R. A.: Treatment of lymphopenic hypogammaglobulinemia and bone-marrow aplasia by transplantation of allogeneic marrow: Crucial role of histocompatibility matching. New Eng. J. Med., 281:691–697, 1969.
62. Miller, M. E.: Thymic dysplasia ("Swiss Agammaglobulinemia"). I. Graft versus host reaction following bone-marrow transfusion. J. Pediat., 70:730–736, 1967.
63. Mitchison, N. A.: Passive transfer of transplantation immunity. Proc. Roy. Soc., B, 142:72–87, 1954.
64. Mitchison, N. A.: Immunologic approaches to cancer. Transplant. Proc., 2:92–103, 1970.
65. Moore, G. E., and Moore, M. B.: Auto-inoculation of cultured human lymphocytes in malignant melanoma. N.Y. State J. Med., 69:460–462, 1969.
66. Nadler, S. H., and Moore, G. E.: Immunotherapy of malignant disease. Arch. Surg., 99:376–381, 1969.
67. O'Connell, C. J., Karzon, D. T., Barron, A. L., Plaut, M. E., and Ali, V. M.: Progressive vaccinia with normal antibodies: A case possibly due to deficient cellular immunity. Ann. Intern. Med., 60:282–289, 1963.
68. Oettgen, H. F., Old, L. J., and Boyse, E. A.: Human tumor immunology. Symposium on Medical Aspects of Cancer. MED. CLIN. N. AMER., 55:761–785, 1971.
69. Oettgen, H., Old, L., Farrow, J., Valentine, F., Lawrence, S., and Thomas, L.: Effects of transfer factor in cancer patients. J. Clin. Invest., 50:71a, Abstr. 239, 1971.
70. Penner, P. E., Cohen, L. H., and Loeb, L. A.: RNA-dependent DNA polymerase in human lymphocytes during gene activation by phytohemagglutinin. Nat. New Biol., 232:58–60, 1971.
71. Plescia, O. J., and Braun, W., eds. Nucleic Acids in Immunology. Proceedings of a Symposium held at the Institute of Microbiology of Rutgers, The State University. New York, Springer Verlag, 1968.
72. Rapaport, F. T., Lawrence, H. S., Millar, J. W., Pappagianis, D., and Smith, C. E.: Transfer of delayed hypersensitivity to coccidioidin in man. J. Immunol., 84:358–367, 1960.
73. Rocklin, R. E., Chilgren, R. A., Hong, R., and David, J. R.: Transfer of cellular hypersensitivity in chronic mucocutaneous candidiasis monitored in vivo and in vitro. Cellular Immunol., 1:290–299, 1970.
74. Rosen, F. S., Gitlin, D., and Janeway, C. A.: Alymphocytosis, agammaglobulinaemia, homografts, and delayed hypersensitivity: Study of a case. Lancet, 2:380–381, 1962.
75. Rosen, F. S., Gotoff, S. P., Craig, J. M., Ritchie, J., and Janeway, C. A.: Further observations on the Swiss type of agammaglobulinemia (Alymphocytosis): The effect of syngeneic bone-marrow cells. New Eng. J. Med., 274:18–21, 1966.
76. Salmon, S. E., Smith, B. A., Lehrer, R. I., Mogerman, S. N., Shinefield, H. R., and Perkins, H. A.: Modification of donor lymphocytes for transplantation in lymphopenic immunological deficiency. Lancet, 2:149–150, 1970.
77. Schulkind, M. L., Adler, W. H., Altemeier, W. A., and Ayoub, E. M.: Transfer factor in the treatment of chronic mucocutaneous candidiasis. Abstracts, American Pediatric Society, Inc., and Society for Pediatric Research, 1971, p. 30.
78. Snell, G. D., Cherry, M., and Démant, P.: Evidence that H-2 private specificities can be arranged in two mutually exclusive systems possibly homologous with two subsystems of HL-A. Transplant. Proc., 3:183–186, 1971.
79. Spitler, L. E., Levin, A. S., Huber, H., and Fudenberg, H. H.: Prediction of results of transfer factor therapy in the Wiskott-Aldrich syndrome by monocyte IgG receptors. Sixth Leucocyte Culture Conference, 1971. New York, Academic Press, to be published.
80. Spitler, L. E., Levin, A. S., Stites, D., Pirofsky, B., and Fudenberg, H. H.: Transfer factor therapy in mucocutaneous candidiasis. Sixth Leucocyte Culture Conference, 1971. New York, Academic Press, to be published.
81. Symes, M. O., Riddell, A. G., Immelman, E. J., and Terblanche, J.: Immunologically competent cells in the treatment of malignant disease. Lancet, 1:1054–1056, 1968.
82. Valentine, F. T., and Lawrence, H. S.: Lymphocyte stimulation: Transfer of cellular hypersensitivity to antigen in vitro. Science, 165:1014–1016, 1969.
83. W.H.O. Committee Report: Primary immunodeficiencies. Pediatrics, 47:927–946, 1971.
84. Wigzell, H., and Andersson, B.: Cell separation on antigen-coated columns. Elimination of high rate antibody-forming cells and immunological memory cells. J. Exper. Med., 129:23–36, 1969.
85. Wolstenholme, G. E. W., and O'Connor, M., eds.: Antilymphocytic Serum. Ciba Foundation Study Group 29. Boston, Little, Brown and Co., 1967.
86. Woodruff, M. F. A., and Nolan, B.: Preliminary observations on treatment of advanced cancer by injection of allogeneic spleen cells. Lancet, 2:426–429, 1963.

Resistance of Guinea Pigs to Leukemia following Transfer of Immunocompetent Allogeneic Lymphoid Cells

David H. Katz, Leonard Ellman, William E. Paul,
Ira Green, and Baruj Benacerraf

SUMMARY

The passive transfer of immunocompetent lymphoid cells from allogeneic strain 13 guinea pigs to normal adult strain 2 recipients which are subsequently challenged with a lethal inoculum of L_2C leukemia significantly alters the development of systemic leukemia in such recipients. This is manifested by striking prolongation of survival times in all allogeneic cell recipients even when doses of L_2C as much as 30-fold higher than the uniformly lethal dose are used. Furthermore, in 21% of all cases long-term protection against development of leukemia has been observed. The temporal relationship between cell transfer and leukemic challenge was shown to be crucial, and the antileukemic protective effect was observed even at a time when all donor cells had presumably been rejected. The primary involvement of host immune mechanisms in this antileukemia protection phenomenon is further suggested by the ability of 50% of allogeneic cell recipients subjected to a second leukemic challenge to reject this lethal L_2C inoculum. We suggest that this protective phenomenon most likely reflects critical cellular actions performed by the host cell population which has been highly stimulated by events related to the graft-*versus*-host reaction. The possible host cell types serving as primary effectors are discussed.

INTRODUCTION

The development of specific tumor immunity has been accomplished in a wide variety of experimental animal tumor systems as a result of immunization with sublethal tumor inocula, inactivated tumor cells, or tumor cell extracts (7, 12, 15, 16, 27). However, a major problem concerns the relatively

129

weak immunogenicity of TSTA.[1] Thus, development of methods to augment the immune response to TSTA may offer a useful approach to the treatment of neoplastic disorders. In this and the accompanying paper (13), we describe one such approach for the development of tumor protection based on the stimulation of host immune mechanisms following induction of a transient GVH reaction.

The utilization of this approach followed from recent studies in our laboratory which demonstrated that the GVH reaction serves as a potent stimulus to certain functions of the immune system. Thus, we found that the transfer of immunocompetent lymphoid cells from inbred donor guinea pigs to allogeneic recipients primed with a hapten-carrier conjugate results in increased synthesis of antihapten and anticarrier antibodies by the recipients in the absence of any further antigenic challenge (18, 19, 21). This phenomenon, which we have termed "allogeneic effect," appears, moreover, to permit direct antigenic stimulation of bone marrow-derived precursors of antibody-forming cells of the host without the cooperative function of thymus-derived, carrier-specific "helper" cells normally required in a variety of humoral immune responses (8, 20, 26, 28).

As reported previously (19, 21), the allogeneic effect is mediated through the existence of a specific immunological response of grafted cells to host cells and does not require the concomitant development of a host rejection reaction against the donor lymphoid cells. These studies demonstrated, therefore, that the GVH reaction serves as a highly potent stimulus to at least certain functions of the immune system. We therefore investigated the feasibility of applying the allogeneic effect phenomenon to stimulate protective immune responses in guinea pigs inoculated with lethal L_2C leukemia.

The L_2C lymphatic leukemia, the only known guinea pig leukemia available for study, arose in an inbred strain 2 guinea pig and has been serially passaged in this strain for the last 17 years (9). We have recently demonstrated the existence of a TSTA on L_2C leukemia cells in that immunization of strain 2 guinea pigs with an aqueous suspension or a CFA emulsion of inactivated tumor cells specifically protects such animals against a lethal inoculum of L_2C leukemia (12). In these studies the presence of specific anti-L_2C antibodies was not detected; rather, the predominant role of cell-mediated immunity in the development of specific resistance to this normally lethal disease was clearly established (12).

[1] The abbreviations used are: TSTA, tumor-specific transplantation antigens; GVH, graft *versus* host; CFA, complete Freund's adjuvant; RES, reticuloendothelial system.

130

In this paper, we show that the passive transfer of immunocompetent allogeneic lymphoid cells to strain 2 guinea pigs prior to administration of a lethal L_2C inoculum results in marked prolongation of survival compared to control guinea pigs which have not received allogeneic cells. Moreover, 21% of strain 2 recipients of allogeneic cells have survived for prolonged periods of observation. The quantity of allogeneic cells used and the temporal relationship between cell transfer and leukemic challenge are shown to be crucial with respect to the ability to prolong survival. Transfer of allogeneic cells exerts a protective effect against a dose of L_2C cells 30-fold higher than the uniformly lethal dose. Finally, the involvement of host immune mechanisms in the protection against leukemia observed in these studies is suggested by the ability of 50% of allogeneic cell recipients to reject a second lethal leukemia cell inoculum. In the accompanying paper (13), we present data concerning the mechanisms involved in this phenomenon.

MATERIALS AND METHODS

Animals. Adult inbred strain 2 and strain 13 guinea pigs weighing 250 to 400 g were obtained from the Division of Research Services, NIH, Bethesda, Md.

Experimental Tumor. Guinea pig L_2C leukemia, a generous gift of Dr. L. S. Kaplow, Yale University School of Medicine, New Haven, Conn., was serially transplanted in our strain 2 guinea pig colony for approximately 14 months. As described in detail elsewhere (12), L_2C cells obtained from the blood of leukemic animals are preserved in 10% dimethyl sulfoxide at $-70°$. Cells stored in this manner retain 70 to 90% viability (by trypan blue exclusion) and normal lethal potency after thawing (12).

Cell Transfers. Strain 13 donor guinea pigs were immunized in the footpads with 0.9% NaCl solution emulsified in CFA (Difco Laboratories, Detroit, Mich.). This was done in order to enlarge the lymph nodes thus increasing the number of lymphocytes obtained. Three weeks later, the animals were killed, and axillary, occipital, inguinal, and popliteal lymph nodes and spleen were removed. Single cell suspensions in Eagle's minimum essential medium were prepared and washed. In general, 1.0×10^9 nucleated cells were transferred i.v. to strain 2 guinea pig recipients.

Statistical Analyses. Survival times after leukemic challenge were logarithmically transformed, and mean and standard errors were calculated. Results from appropriate groups were compared by Student's t test.

131

RESULTS

Course of L_2C Leukemia in Untreated Strain 2 Guinea Pigs

As reported elsewhere (12), a rather characteristic clinical course is observed in normal strain 2 guinea pigs inoculated intradermally with 0.3×10^6 L_2C leukemia cells. Briefly, a hemorrhagic, nodular leukemic tumor appears at the intradermal injection site 7 to 14 days after inoculation. Seven to 10 days later, progressive systemic disease is manifested by striking leukocytosis (300,000 to 400,000 white cells/cu mm), abdominal distention with palpable hepatosplenomegaly, marked ataxia, and shortly thereafter death. Gross autopsy examination reveals massive hepatosplenomegaly and enlarged lymph nodes and thymus.

Effect of Passive Transfer of Immunocompetent Allogeneic Lymphoid Cells on the Survival of Strain 2 Guinea Pigs Challenged with Leukemia

The initial experiment was designed to determine whether stimulation of host immune mechanisms by the allogeneic effect phenomenon, with properties as described under "Introduction," would appreciably influence the response of strain 2 guinea pigs to a highly lethal dose of L_2C leukemia cells.

Lymph node and spleen cells (1.0×10^9) from strain 13 guinea pig donors were injected i.v. into normal allogeneic strain 2 recipients. Six days after allogeneic cell transfer, 0.3 to 0.4×10^6 L_2C leukemia cells were administered intradermally to individual recipient guinea pigs and to control strain 2 guinea pigs which had not received allogeneic cells. All animals were then observed for development of local intradermal tumor nodules at the site of inoculation and for signs of systemic disease.

In the studies reported in this and the accompanying paper (13), we present the data in terms of the interval between intradermal inoculation of leukemia cells and death of individual control and experimental guinea pigs, irrespective of whether or not the occurrence of leukemia in a given animal was evident at gross autopsy examination. Where applicable, the number of animals in a given group with no evidence of leukemia at death will be noted in the chart legends and the text. Furthermore, the mean survival times and standard errors presented were calculated only on the basis of deaths that occurred in given experiments; surviving animals are presented separately.

Survival times after the L_2C leukemic challenge of control strain 2 guinea pigs and strain 2 recipients of 1×10^9 allogeneic strain 13 lymphoid cells are summarized in Chart 1.

Individual deaths in both groups as well as geometric mean survival and standard errors are illustrated. A very striking and highly significant prolongation of survival time was observed among the experimental animals given allogeneic lymphoid cells 6 days before the leukemic challenge as compared to the nontreated controls (0.001 $> p$). There were 70 control guinea pigs, all of which died during the course of the experiment. Sixty-nine deaths were attributable to systemic leukemia as evidenced by development of leukemic skin tumors, abdominal distention and organomegaly, and terminal ataxia. The remaining control guinea pig died on Day 17 after challenge with no gross evidence of systemic leukemia.

Of 38 animals in the experimental group, 30 died during the period of observation; the results are presented in Chart 1. Twenty-four of the 30 guinea pigs that died clearly succumbed as a result of systemic leukemia despite the fact that one-third of these animals had not developed leukemic skin tumors prior to death. The remaining 6 animals in this group had no detectable gross pathological lesions at autopsy characteristic of guinea pig leukemia and, moreover, had never developed leukemic skin tumors during their course. The mean survival time of the experimental animals that died was significantly prolonged as a result of the allogeneic cell transfer.

At the termination of these experiments, and indeed at the time of preparation of this manuscript, 21% of the experimental guinea pigs that received strain 13 allogeneic lymphoid cells 6 days prior to leukemia cell inoculation are still alive and healthy. Thus, 8 of 38 strain 2 recipients of strain 13 cells have survived for periods ranging from 80 to 150 days after initial leukemic challenge and have no evidence of systemic disease or skin tumors. There are no survivors among the 70 control guinea pigs.

Capacity to Prolong Survival of Strain 2 Guinea Pigs Challenged with Leukemia as a Result of Transfer of Allogeneic Strain 13 Lymphoid Cells

Relationship of Time Interval between Cell Transfer and Leukemia Challenge. The preceding experiment demonstrates clearly that transfer of immunocompetent lymphoid cells from allogeneic strain 13 guinea pigs into strain 2 guinea pig recipients significantly modifies the responses of such recipients to a normally lethal dose of L_2C leukemia cells administered 6 days after cell transfer. Our earlier investigations on the stimulation of antibody responses by the allogeneic effect demonstrated that a critical time relationship exists between transfer of allogeneic cells and secondary antigen administration (19, 21). We therefore felt that a

133

detailed study of the relationship of timing between allogeneic cell transfer and leukemic challenge and the capacity to prolong survival in allogeneic cell recipients would provide some insight into the kinetics of cellular events in this phenomenon.

Normal strain 2 guinea pigs were given i.v. injections of 1 X 10^9 lymph node and spleen cells from allogeneic strain 13 donor guinea pigs. Allogeneic cell recipients and normal strain 2 control animals were then given intradermal inoculations of 0.3 X 10^6 L_2C leukemia cells at various time intervals after cell transfer.

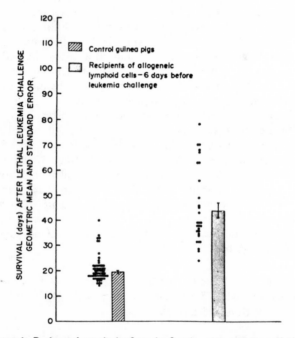

Chart 1. Prolonged survival of strain 2 guinea pigs challenged with lethal leukemia following passive transfer of immunocompetent allogeneic lymphoid cells. Lymph node and spleen cells (1.0 X 10^9) from strain 13 donor guinea pigs were injected i.v. into individual allogeneic strain 2 recipients. Six days later, 38 allogeneic cell recipients and 70 control strain 2 guinea pigs that had not received allogeneic cells were given inoculations intradermally of 0.3 to 0.4 X 10^6 L_2C leukemia cells. Individual deaths in both groups as well as geometric mean survival times and S.E. are illustrated. Eight of 38 allogeneic cell recipients are still alive and are therefore not included in this chart. A comparison of the geometric mean survival time of allogeneic cell recipients with that of control guinea pigs yielded a p value of <0.001.

134

In the 1st experiment, 6 strain 2 recipients in 1 group were challenged with leukemia cells within 5 minutes after receiving the allogeneic lymphoid cells, while 6 recipients in a 2nd group received their leukemic challenge 6 days after cell transfer. The results of this experiment, illustrated in Chart 2, demonstrate again the very striking prolongation of survival in recipients challenged with leukemia 6 days after allogeneic cell transfer as compared to nontransferred controls ($0.001 > p$). In contrast, survival time of allogeneic cell recipients given their leukemic challenge on the same day as the cell transfer was only modestly increased over that of controls ($0.02 > p > 0.01$).

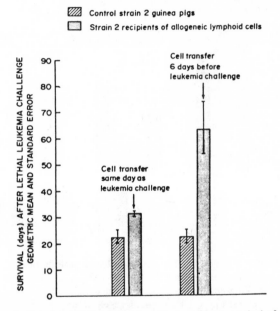

Chart 2. Relationship between capacity to prolong survival of strain 2 guinea pigs challenged with lethal leukemia and the time interval between allogeneic cell transfer and leukemic challenge. Lymph node and spleen cells (1.0×10^9) from allogeneic strain 13 donor guinea pigs were injected i.v. into normal strain 2 recipients. Six recipients in 1 group were given intradermal inoculations of 0.3 to 0.4×10^6 L_2C cells immediately after cell transfer, while 6 recipients in a 2nd group received their leukemic challenge 6 days after cell transfer. Geometric mean survival times and S.E. of the 2 experimental groups and of 8 control strain 2 guinea pigs are illustrated. A comparison of the geometric mean survival times of the experimental and control groups gave the following results. Comparison of controls with allogeneic recipients challenged on the same day yielded a p value of $0.02 > p > 0.01$. Comparison of controls with allogeneic cell recipients challenged 6 days after transfer yielded a p value of <0.001.

135

In the 2nd experiment, groups consisting of 4 to 5 strain 2 recipients were challenged with leukemia cells at an interval of either 1, 3, 6, 13, or 21 days after allogeneic cell transfer. The allogeneic cell transfers were scheduled so that all groups of recipient guinea pigs and 1 group of 4 normal control guinea pigs received their leukemic challenges on the same day from the same aliquot of L_2C cells. The results of this study are presented in Chart 3. Survival times were clearly prolonged in strain 2 recipients of allogeneic strain 13 cells which were challenged with leukemia cells at an interval of either 1, 3, 6, or 13 days after cell transfer. The highest levels of significance ($0.001 > p$), when compared to control survival times, were

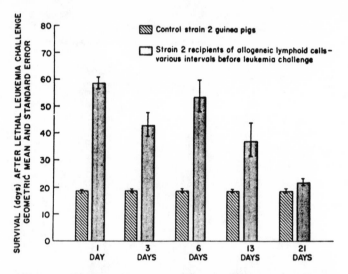

Chart 3. Relationship between capacity to prolong survival of strain 2 guinea pigs challenged with lethal leukemia and the time interval between allogeneic cell transfer and leukemic challenge. Lymph node and spleen cells (1×10^9) from allogeneic strain 13 donor guinea pigs were injected i.v. into normal strain 2 recipients. Groups of 4 to 5 recipients were given intradermal inoculations of 0.3 to 0.4 $\times$ 10^6 L_2C cells at an interval of either 1, 3, 6, 13, or 21 days after cell transfer. Geometric mean survival times and S.E. of the 5 experimental groups and of 1 group of 4 control strain 2 guinea pigs are illustrated.

A comparison of the geometric mean survival times of the control group with each experimental group gave the following results. Comparison of the controls with the 1-, 3-, and 6-day interval recipient groups yielded a p value of <0.001 in each case. Comparison of the controls with the 13- and 21-day interval recipient groups yielded p values of $0.02 > p > 0.01$ and $0.10 > p > 0.05$, respectively. Similar comparisons among the experimental groups gave the following results. Comparison of the 21-day interval group with the other recipient groups yielded the following p values: (a) 1-day, $p < 0.001$; (b) 3-day, $p < 0.001$; (c) 6-day, $p < 0.001$; (d) 13-day, $0.02 > p > 0.01$.

136

attained in the 1-, 3-, and 6-day interval groups. Allogeneic cell recipients challenged 13 days after transfer attained moderately prolonged survival times of slightly lesser significance compared to controls $(0.02 > p > 0.01)$ than those of the 1-, 3-, and 6-day groups. The survival times of allogeneic cell recipients challenged 21 days after transfer were not significantly prolonged over those of control guinea pigs $(0.10 > p > 0.05)$ and, moreover, were considerably lower than survival times of the 1-, 3-, and 6-day recipient groups $(0.001 > p)$ and those of the 13-day recipients $(0.02 > p > 0.01)$.

These experiments indicate, therefore, that the capacity to prolong survival of guinea pigs with leukemia as a result of a single allogeneic cell transfer bears a crucial relationship to the time interval between cell transfer and administration of the lethal leukemia inoculum. Thus, transfer of allogeneic cells 21 days prior to leukemic challenge is completely ineffective in prolonging survival, and when allogeneic cells are transferred immediately prior to challenge, survival times are prolonged only slightly. Survival is moderately prolonged in recipient guinea pigs challenged with leukemia 13 days after allogeneic cell transfer, whereas survival times are markedly prolonged in guinea pigs receiving allogeneic cells 1, 3, or 6 days before leukemia inoculation.

Effect of Varying the Number of Passively Transferred Allogeneic Lymphoid Cells on the Prolongation of Survival Times of Guinea Pigs Challenged with Leukemia. Individual normal strain 2 guinea pig recipients were given i.v. injections with either 50×10^6, 200×10^6, or 1000×10^6 lymph node and spleen cells from allogeneic strain 13 donors which had been immunized 3 weeks previously with 0.9% NaCl solution emulsified in CFA. Six days after cell transfer, all recipients and 1 group of normal strain 2 control guinea pigs were given intradermal inoculations of 0.3 to 0.4×10^6 L_2C leukemia cells and then observed for development of systemic diseases.

The results of this experiment, illustrated in Chart 4, demonstrate a highly significant prolongation of survival times in strain 2 recipients of 1000×10^6 strain 13 lymphoid cells as compared to controls $(0.001 > p)$. On the other hand, survival times were only moderately prolonged in recipients of 200×10^6 allogeneic cells, and no significant effect was observed in recipients of 50×10^6 allogeneic cells. Thus, the greatest degree of protection occurs when 1000×10^6 donor cells are used.

Effect of Varying the Dose of L_2C Leukemia Cells Administered.

Lymph node and spleen cells (1.0×10^9) from strain 13 donors were injected i.v. into individual normal strain 2 recipients. Six days after allogeneic cell transfers, 4 groups of recipients and 4 groups of normal control strain 2 guinea pigs were given intradermal inoculations of either 0.3×10^6, 1.0×10^6, 3.0×10^6, or 6.0×10^6 L_2C leukemia cells. All recipient and control animals were then followed closely for evidence of systemic disease.

As illustrated in Chart 5, allogeneic cell recipients challenged with either 0.3, 1.0, or 3.0 $\times 10^6$ L_2C cells attained significantly prolonged survival times compared to their respective groups. Survival times of recipients challenged with 6.0 $\times 10^6$ L_2C cells were prolonged, although to a somewhat lesser degree of significance when compared to their controls. As reported elsewhere (12), 0.1×10^6 L_2C leukemia cells administered intradermally is a uniformly lethal dose in strain 2 guinea pigs. In this experiment, significantly prolonged survival times were obtained, as a result of allogeneic cell

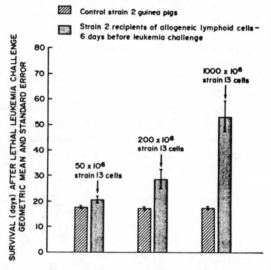

Chart 4. Effect of varying the number of transferred allogeneic cells on the prolongation of survival times of strain 2 guinea pigs challenged with lethal leukemia. Individual strain 2 recipients were given i.v. injections of either 50×10^6, 200×10^6 or $1,000 \times 10^6$ lymph node and spleen cells from allogeneic strain 13 donor guinea pigs. Six days after cell transfer, the 4 recipients in each experimental group were given intradermal inoculations of 0.3 to 0.4×10^6 L_2C cells. Geometric mean survival times and S.E. of the 3 experimental groups and of 1 group of 4 control strain 2 guinea pigs are illustrated. A comparison of the control group with each experimental group gave the following results. Comparison of the controls with the recipients of 50×10^6 cells and of 200×10^6 cells yielded p values of $0.05 > p > 0.025$ and $0.01 > p > 0.005$, respectively. Comparison of the controls with recipients of 1000×10^6 cells yielded a p value of <0.001.

transfer, in guinea pigs challenged with a dose of leukemia cells at least 30 times larger than the uniformly lethal dose in untreated animals.

Response of Strain 2 Guinea Pigs Previously Protected against Leukemia As a Result of Allogeneic Cell Transfer to a Second Leukemic Challenge. The experiments described thus far have demonstrated the ability to markedly alter the normal development of systemic leukemia in strain 2 guinea pigs as a result of the passive transfer of immunocompetent allogeneic lymphoid cells prior to leukemic challenge. This is reflected by a significant prolongation of survival times in essentially all cases and by what appears to be either prevention or permanent remission in 21% of such recipients. One crucial question is whether tumor-specific immunity has developed in these survivors which may be effective in affording long-term

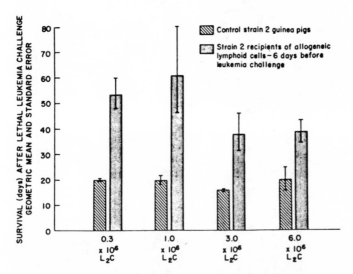

Chart 5. Effect of varying the dose of the L_2C cell challenge on the capacity to prolong survival of strain 2 guinea pigs as a result of allogeneic cell transfer. Lymph node and spleen cells (1.0×10^9) from strain 13 donor guinea pigs were injected i.v. into individual allogeneic strain 2 recipients. Six days after cell transfer, 4 groups consisting of 4 recipients each and 4 groups of 3 control strain 2 guinea pigs were given intradermal inoculations of either 0.3×10^6, 1.0×10^6, 3.0×10^6, or 6.0×10^6 L_2C cells. Geometric mean survival times and S.E. of each experimental and control group are illustrated. A comparison of the geometric mean survival times of each experimental group of recipients with their respective controls gave the following results: (a) 0.3×10^6 dose, $0.005 > p > 0.001$; (b) 1.0×10^6 dose, $0.02 > p > 0.01$; (c) 3.0×10^6 dose, $0.01 > p > 0.05$; (d) 6.0×10^6 dose, $0.05 > p > 0.025$.

139

Table 1

Response of strain 2 guinea pig recipients of allogeneic lymphoid cells to a second lethal dose of L_2C leukemia cells

Recipient guinea pigs were given i.v. injections of 1×10^9 allogeneic strain 13 lymph node and spleen cells 6 days before the first intradermal inoculation, in the doses indicated, of L_2C leukemia cells. The recipients listed here, which had survived the initial leukemic challenge for varying lengths of time, as shown above, with no evidence of systemic leukemia were subjected to a second intradermal inoculation of 3.0×10^6 L_2C cells. Control animals (not shown) inoculated at the same time with 3.0×10^6 L_2C cells survived 16, 19, and 20 days, respectively.

Animal	First dose of L_2C cells ($\times 10^6$)	Days survived at time of rechallenge with L_2C	Days survived after rechallenge with L_2C	Length of survival (days) after rechallenge as of June 11, 1971
1	0.3	99	21	
2	0.3	63	18	
3	3.0	63	21	
4	3.0	63	46	
5	0.3	63	Still alive	88
6	0.3	56	Still alive	88
7	0.3	22	Still alive	101
8	0.3	22	Still alive	101

140

or perhaps permanent protection against the leukemia. To approach this point, 8 strain 2 recipients of allogeneic cells which had survived for varying lengths of time after initial lethal leukemic challenge, without discernible evidence of systemic disease, were subjected to a 2nd leukemic challenge consisting of a 10-fold higher dose (3.0×10^6) of L_2C cells.

Details on these 8 guinea pigs and their course subsequent to the second leukemic challenge are presented in Table 1. Control guinea pigs given inoculations of 3.0×10^6 L_2C cells at the time when the experimental animals were rechallenged survived for 16, 19, and 20 days, respectively. Of the experimental animals, 3 were clearly no different from the controls, surviving 18, 21, and 21 days, respectively. A 4th recipient survived significantly longer (46 days) but, nevertheless, succumbed with systemic leukemia. In contrast, 4 of the recipient guinea pigs have survived for very long periods after the second leukemic challenge and appear, in all respects, to be vigorous and healthy. It appears likely, therefore, that protective tumor-specific immunity has developed in one-half of the allogeneic cell recipients subjected to rechallenge. In this regard, in 2 of the 4 recipients surviving rechallenge, we observed the development of small leukemic skin tumors approximately 7 to 10 days after rechallenge and the subsequent rejection and disappearance of these lesions within 5 to 8 days.

DISCUSSION

The studies presented here have shown that the course of lethal L_2C leukemia in inbred strain 2 guinea pigs is significantly altered as a result of the passive transfer of immunocompetent allogeneic lymphoid cells. This is manifested by striking prolongation of survival times in essentially all such recipients even when doses of L_2C cells as much as 30-fold higher than the uniformly lethal dose are used. Moreover, in 21% of all cases long-term protection against development of leukemia has been observed. The allogeneic cell transfer was the only form of treatment used in these experiments. None of the experimental animals were subjected to either X-irradiation or cytotoxic drug therapy. The occurrence of acute toxic sequelae attributable to such therapeutic modes and the development of acute or chronic GVH reactions as a result of allogeneic cell transfer were thus avoided as complicating features in this system.

The use of foreign hematopoietic cells as a therapeutic

approach against leukemia or other neoplastic disorders is by no means novel. Thus, independent investigators have used immunocompetent allogeneic or xenogeneic cells in models of murine leukemia (1, 3–5, 23, 29), other transplantable mouse tumors (11, 31–33), and, in some instances, advanced human neoplasms (6, 14, 22, 24, 30). In general, however, the studies cited differ from the system described in this paper in that total body X-irradiation, cytotoxic drugs, or both were important features in the experimental design. Typically, mice with leukemia or solid tumors were lethally or sublethally irradiated prior to injection of allogeneic or xenogeneic lymphoid cells. This regimen usually resulted in a high mortality among experimental animals due to either acute radiation syndrome, acute GVH reaction, or chronic GVH reaction. Modifying this regimen by including cytotoxic drug therapy against the adverse effects of the GVH reaction has led to significantly prolonged survival of radiation chimeras without recurrence of leukemia (3).

With human cancers, temporary remissions in some patients with chemotherapy-resistant acute leukemias following transfusions of leukocytes from patients with chronic myelogenous leukemia have been described by Mathé et al. (24). There appeared to be an excellent correlation between remission of leukemia and the appearance of signs of the GVH reaction. Transplantation of allogeneic bone marrow into terminal leukemia patients who had been treated with ablative doses of X-irradiation or cyclophosphamide has led to apparent eradication of the leukemia in a few instances, although the patients succumbed to GVH disease (6, 14, 22).

The interpretations of these investigators regarding tumor suppression following such allogeneic or xenogeneic cell transfers include: (a) allogeneic inhibition; (b) overgrowth of tumor cells, the proliferation rate of which may have been diminished following irradiation, by more rapidly dividing allogeneic or xenogeneic cells; (c) destruction of tumor cells, bearing identical histo-compatibility specificities as the normal host cells, by the GVH response of the transferred allogeneic immunocompetent cells; or (d) destruction of tumor cells by donor cells which have become specifically sensitized against tumor-specific transplantation antigens. These various explanations all imply that the antitumor effect of the GVH reaction is achieved through actions of the allogeneic donor cells on the tumor tissue.

In these studies, a crucial temporal relationship was found to exist between the transfer of allogeneic cells and the administration of the lethal leukemia inoculum. Thus, highly significant protection was observed in guinea pigs that received the allogeneic lymphoid cells 1, 3, or 6 days prior to lethal

142

leukemic challenge. The protective effect was diminished somewhat in the cases where 13 days elapsed between cell transfer and leukemic challenge. In sharp contrast, transfer of allogeneic cells 21 days prior to leukemic challenge was completely ineffective in prolonging survival times, and when allogeneic cells were transferred immediately prior to challenge, only slightly prolonged survival times were observed.

When considering which cells of the host are primarily responsible for the antileukemic effect, there are essentially but 2 realistic possibilities: (a) the primary phagocytic cells of the RES, i.e., macrophages; and (b) the immunocompetent lymphocyte. It has been well established by others working with mice and rats that during the 3rd week following induction of the GVH reaction in nonirradiated F_1 recipients of parental donor cells, there is a significant increase in resistance to bacterial infection (2, 10). This has been attributed to heightened activation of the host macrophage population which has been shown to occur by the 2nd or 3rd week of the GVH response (17). It might reasonably be expected that sufficient numbers of such highly activated cells in the RES of the host could exert a nonspecific antitumor cell effect. Indeed, Medzihradsky (25), working with a transplantable tumor in rats, interpreted a modest antitumor effect he observed in this way. In his system, prolonged survival was attained in F_1 recipients of parental cells transferred 14 days prior to tumor inoculation. Shorter or longer intervals between cell transfer and tumor challenge were ineffective. He suggested that the proliferation of host RES cells during the GVH reaction was responsible for this effect. In contrast, optimal antileukemic effects in our system occur much earlier in the course of the GVH response. The diminished protection observed in guinea pigs challenged with L_2C cells 13 days after allogeneic cell transfer and the failure to obtain antileukemic effects 21 days after transfer would argue against a primary role for hyperactive macrophages in this phenomenon. Nevertheless, a major role for these and other cells of the RES cannot be excluded.

These results are enlightening in the context of cellular kinetics in this phenomenon in that the transferred donor cells, themselves fully immunocompetent and thereby capable of reacting specifically against host tissues, are transplanted into a foreign environment consisting of similarly immunocompetent host lymphoid cells which not only possess full capacity to reject the donor cells but maintain a decided advantage in numbers as well. In this circumstance, we may therefore assume that essentially all allogeneic donor cells are rejected by the recipient in relatively short order. Assuming, as we have, that the 6-day interval between cell transfer and L_2C challenge is optimal, it would seem very unlikely that sufficient numbers of donor cells, if any at all, are present in a fully functional state with the capacity to reject directly the inoculated L_2C cells. The same reasoning in reverse, on the other hand, would make a reasonable argument that in the cases of the 1-day or even, perhaps, the 3-day interval recipients, sufficient numbers of viable, functional donor cells may exist to recognize and reject the foreign leukemic cells in the absence of active participation of host cells. However, if that were the case, the same effect should be true when allogeneic cells are transferred immediately prior to leukemic challenge, and this was not observed. The more appealing and perhaps more likely explanation is that the critical cellular events in the expression of the protective phenomenon are ultimately performed by the host cell population which has been highly stimulated, in an as yet undefined manner, by the GVH reaction.

Evidence that the ultimate role is performed by host cells will be presented in the accompanying paper (13). Hence, we demonstrate that protection against L_2C leukemia in this system requires the development of the GVH reaction in lymphoid organs of the host as evidenced by the failure to observe such protection in strain 2 recipients of semisyngeneic 2×13 F_1 hybrid donor cells. The ineffectiveness of 2×13 F_1 lymphoid cells in affording antileukemia protection demonstrates that more than just antigenic stimulation of host cells is involved in the mediation of this effect. Furthermore, we show that passive transfer of parental strain 2 or strain 13 lymphoid cells into 2×13 F_1 recipients, which are genetically incapable of rejecting the parental donor cells, protects such recipients against the L_2C leukemia (13). This latter finding clearly demonstrates that the phenomenon depends solely on the existence of a GVH reaction and does not require the concomitant development of a host rejection response against donor lymphoid cells. The fact that parental strain 2 lymphoid cells are equivalent to strain 13 lymphoid cells in affording protection against leukemia in 2×13 F_1 recipients (13) definitively excludes the possibility that donor cells directly reject the L_2C leukemia on the basis of an immune response directed at strain 2 histocompatibility antigens present on L_2C cells.

One is left then to consider that the population of immunologically competent lymphocytes of the host plays the crucial role in antileukemia protection. Our previous experience with the allogeneic effect phenomenon concerning humoral immune responses shows clearly that very striking stimulatory events on such cells do occur during the GVH

144

reaction (18, 19, 21). Moreover, it appears that immunological memory as well as antibody synthesis may be heightened as a result of this phenomenon (19). It is reasonable to postulate that, in a similar way, immunocompetent host lymphoid cells are highly stimulated, as a result of the GVH reaction, to serve as effectors in specific immune responses against the L_2C leukemia cells. The demonstration that persistent tumor immunity against the L_2C cells existed in one-half of the allogeneic cell recipients subjected to rechallenge argues in favor of this hypothesis. The following report will consider these and other possibilities in greater detail (13).

ACKNOWLEDGMENTS

We gratefully acknowledge the expert technical assistance of Miss Lula Jackson, Mr. Robert McClesky, Mrs. Clara Horton, Mr. Charles Hoes, and Mrs. Susan Pickeral.

REFERENCES

1. Barnes, D. W. H., and Loutit, J. F. Treatment of Murine Leukemia with X-rays and Homologous Bone Marrow. Brit. J. Haematol. *3:* 241–252, 1957.
2. Blanden, R. V. Increased Antibacterial Resistance and Immunodepression during Graft-*versus*-Host Reactions in Mice. Transplantation, *7:* 484-497, 1969.
3. Boranić, M. Transient Graft-*versus*-Host Reaction in the Treatment of Leukemia in Mice. J. Natl. Cancer Inst., *41:* 421–433. 1968.
4. Boranić, M. Delayed Mortality of Sublethally Irradiated Mice Treated with Allogeneic Lymphoid and Myeloid Cells. J. Natl. Cancer Inst., *41:* 439–450, 1968.
5. Boranić, M. Transplantability of Leukemia from Leukemic Mice after Irradiation and Injection of Allogeneic Spleen Cells. European J. Clin. Biol. Res., *15:* 104–109, 1970.
6. Buckner, C. D., Epstein, R. B., Rudolph, R. H., Cleft, R. A., Storb, R., and Thomas, E. D. Allogeneic Marrow Engraftment following Whole Body Irradiation in a Patient with Leukemia. Blood, *35:* 741–750, 1970.
7. Churchill, W. H., Jr., Rapp, H. J., Kronman, B. S., and Borsos, T. Detection of Antigens of a New Diethylnitrosamine-induced Transplantable Hepatoma by Delayed Hypersensitivity. J. Natl. Cancer Inst., *41:* 13–29, 1968.
8. Claman, H. N., and Chaperon, E. A. Immunologic Complementation between Thymus and Marrow Cells—A Model for the Two-Cell Theory of Immunocompetence. Transplantation Rev., *1:* 92–113, 1969.
9. Congdon, C. C., and Lorenz, E. Leukemia in Guinea Pigs. Am. J. Pathol., *30:* 337–359, 1954.
10. Cooper, G. N., and Howard, J. G. An Effect of the Graft-*Versus*-Host Reaction on Resistance to Experimental Bacteremia. Brit. J. Exptl. Pathol., *42:* 558–563, 1961.

145

11. DeVries, M. J., and Vos, O. Treatment of Murine Lymphosarcoma by Total Body X-irradiation and by Injection of Bone Marrow and Lymph Node Cells. J. Natl. Cancer Inst., 21: 1117–1129, 1959.
12. Ellman, L., and Green, I. L$_2$C Guinea Pig Leukemia: Immunoprotection and Immunotherapy. Cancer, in press.
13. Ellman, L., Katz, D. H., Green, I., Paul, W. E., and Benacerraf, B. Mechanisms Involved in the Antileukemic Effect of Allogeneic Lymphoid Cell Transfer. Cancer Res., 32: 141–148, 1972.
14. Graw, R. G., Herzig, G. P., Rogentine, G. N., Yankee, R. A., Levanthal, B., Whang-Peng, J., Halterman, R. H., Kruger, G., Berardi, C., and Henderson, E.S. Graft-versus-Host Reaction Complicating HLA-matched Bone-Marrow Transplantation. Lancet, 2: 1053–1055, 1970.
15. Gross, L. Intradermal Immunization of C$_3$H Mice against a Sarcoma That Originated in an Animal of the Same Line. Cancer Res., 3: 326–333, 1943.
16. Holmes, E. C., Kahan, B. D., and Morton, D. L. Soluble Tumor Specific Transplantation Antigens from Methylcholanthrene-induced Guinea Pig Sarcomas. Cancer, 25: 373–380, 1970.
17. Howard, J. G. Changes in the Activity of the Reticuloendothelial System (RES) following the Injection of Parental Spleen Cells in F$_1$ Hybrid Mice. Brit. J. Exptl. Pathol., 42: 72–82, 1961.
18. Katz, D. H., Davie, J. M., Paul, W. E., and Benacerraf, B. Carrier Function in Anti-hapten Antibody Responses. IV. Experimental Conditions for the Induction of Hapten-specific Tolerance or for the Stimulation of Antihapten Anamnestic Responses by "Non-immunogenic" Hapten Polypeptide Conjugates. J. Exptl. Med., 134: 201–223, 1971.
19. Katz, D. H., Paul, W. E., and Benacerraf, B. Carrier Function in Anti-hapten Antibody Responses. V. Analysis of Cellular Events in the Enhancement of Antibody Responses by the "Allogeneic Effect" in DNP-OVA Primed Guinea Pigs Challenged with a Heterologous DNP-Conjugate. J. Immunol., 107: 1319–1328, 1971.
20. Katz, D. H., Paul, W. E., Goidl, E. A., and Benacerraf, B. Carrier Function in Anti-hapten Immune Responses. I. Enhancement of Primary and Secondary Anti-hapten Antibody Responses by Carrier Preimmunization. J. Exptl. Med., 132: 261–282, 1970.
21. Katz, D. H., Paul, W. E., Goidl, E. A., and Benacerraf, B. Carrier Function in Anti-hapten Antibody Responses. III. Stimulation of Antibody Synthesis and Facilitation of Hapten-specific Secondary Antibody Responses by Graft-versus-Host Reactions. J. Exptl. Med., 133: 169–186, 1971.
22. Mathé, G., Amiel, J. L., Schwarzenberg, L., Catton, A., Schneider, M., DeVries, M. J., Tubina, M., Lalanne, C. L., Binet, J. L., Paprenik, M., Sesman, G., Matsukura, M., Mery, A. M., Schwarzman, V., and Flaister, A. Successful Allogeneic Bone Marrow Transplantation in Man: Chimerism, Induced Specific Tolerance, and Possible Anti-leukemic Effects. Blood 25: 179–196, 1965.
23. Mathé, G., and Bernard, J. Essais de Traitement de la Leucemie Greffe 1210 par l'Irradiation X Suivie de Transfusion de Cellules

Hematopoitque Normales (Isologoues ou Homologoues Myeloides ou Lymphoides, Adultes ou Embryonaires). Rev. Franc. Etud. Clin. Biol., *4:* 442–446, 1959.

24. Mathé, G., Schwarzenberg, L., Amiel, J. L., Pouillart, P., Schneider, M., and Catton, A. Experimental Basis and Clinical Results of Leukemia Adoptive Immunotherapy. Recent Advan. Cancer Res., *30:* 76–84, 1970.

25. Medzihradsky, J. Modification of Tumor Homograft Immunity during the Graft-*versus*-Host Reaction. Neoplasma, *13:* 223–226, 1966.

26. Mitchison, N. A., Rajewsky, K., and Taylor, R. B. Cooperation of Antigenic Determinants and of Cells in the Induction of Antibodies. *In:* J. Šterzl and H. Říha (eds.), Developmental Aspects of Antibody Formation and Structure. Prague: Academia Publishing House of the Czechoslovak Academy of Sciences, 547–553, 1970.

27. Oettgen, H. F., Old, L. J., McLean, E. P., and Carswell, E. A. Delayed Hypersensitivity and Transplantation Immunity Elicited by Soluble Antigens of Chemically Induced Tumors in Inbred Guinea Pigs. Nature, *220:* 295–297, 1968.

28. Rajewsky, K., Schirrmacher, V., Nase, S., and Jerne, N. K. The Requirement of More Than One Antigenic Determinant for Immunogenicity. J. Exptl. Med., *129:* 1131–1143, 1969.

29. Wallis, V., Davies, A. J. S., and Koller, P. C. Inhibition of Radiation-induced Leukemia by the Injection of Hematopoietic Tissue: A Study of Chimerism. Nature, *210:* 500–504, 1966.

30. Woodruff, M. F. A., and Nolan, B. Preliminary Observations on Treatment of Advanced Cancer by Injection of Allogeneic Spleen Cells. Lancet, *2:* 426–429, 1963.

31. Woodruff, M. F. A., and Symes, M. O. The Use of Immunologically Competent Cells in the Treatment of Cancer. Brit. J. Cancer *16:* 707–715, 1962.

32. Woodruff, M. F. A., Symes, M. O., and Anderson, N. F. The Effect of Intraperitoneal Injection of Thoracic Duct Lymphocytes from Normal and Immunized Rats in Mice Inoculated with the Landschutz Ascites Tumor. Brit. J. Cancer, *17:* 482–486, 1963.

33. Woodruff, M. F. A., Symes, M. O., and Stuart, A. E. The Effect of Rat Spleen Cells on Two Transplanted Mouse Tumors. Brit. J. Cancer, *17:* 320–327, 1963.

147

Immunologic Approach to Cancer

N. A. Mitchison

When I started work in George Snell's laboratory at Bar Harbor in 1953, we were all deeply involved in tumor work. George's own little group was busy using genetics to explore and define the transplantation antigens; at that time we were only just beginning to feel justified in referring to them as antigens, and George himself, if I remember correctly, still preferred the more neutral term "factor." Next door, Nat Kaliss was working out the biology of enhancement, and Eugene Day had started up the quest for a purified transplantation antigen. Pancho Hoecker arrived at the same time as I did. He brought the serological skills which he had just acquired in England and started applying them to George's newly-defined antigens, and I tried to do the same for cellular immunity.

Although we were all using tumors in our work one way or another, none of us was really engaged with the immunologic problem of cancer in the strict sense; we were thoroughly skeptical. We knew, of course, that the theory had been proposed that tumor cells bear specific antigens (hereafter referred to as TSA) which are not present on normal cells and that the immune response to these antigens might enable an individual to reject a tumor. We were put off this theory by several things, among which perhaps the strongest was the fact that it already had such a long, checkered, and utterly inconclusive history. We read Woglom's 23-year-old review, and we felt that all the effort which had been expended since then hadn't taken matters any further. We felt that the research which we were engaged in was triumphantly vindicat-

149

ing Woglom's standpoint, which was that tumor cells carry powerful transplantation antigens and nothing else. We also felt that George's genetics were uncovering a magnificent array of varied transplantation antigens, so numerous that they could easily account for all the phenomena of rejection of tumor transplants, even when these occurred within nominally inbred strains of mice or rats.

It took me a long time to admit I was wrong. In 1960 I read a skeptical paper at the opening of the new cancer research building at Berkeley. Actually it was a rotten paper and I felt miserable afterward. In retrospect I would like to think that this was because of my guilt at neglecting the evidence in favor of TSA. After all, Prehn and Main's classical paper[1] on immunity to methylcholanthrene-induced sarcomas was already two years old. No doubt I wanted to underrate their work because it did not involve isotopes, and just then I was learning how radically they could change the practice of immunology.

Let me then use the present occasion to look again at the tumor antigen problem. If one dismisses choriocarcinoma as a very special case involving alloantigens, there are two types of tumor which clearly display TSA: tumors induced in laboratory animals by chemicals and by viruses. The strongest evidence of an effective immune response to TSA in these cases comes from the demonstration of protective immunization against the tumor. Immunization can be obtained fairly easily with graded cell doses, killed cells, or surgical resection of a growing tumor. Less frequently immunization can also be obtained with cell extracts and by passive immunization with serum or adoptive immunization with cells. In general, immunity to TSA parallels immunity to alloantigens. For example, only lymphoid or marrow tumors are susceptible to destruction by antiserum; the more solid tumors are susceptible rather to cell-mediated immunity.

With other animal tumors a response to TSA can be demonstrated only with difficulty, if at all. In particular, spontaneous tumors, not known to be of viral origin, usually do not display TSA. The generalization runs that the longer the latent period of a tumor, the weaker is its antigenicity. This trend has usually been interpreted as evidence of immunoselection during the development of late tumors in favor of more weakly antigenic variants. Tumors in man also differ widely in their ability to evoke a detectable immune response, with Burkitt's lymphoma and melanoma at the strong end of the range. The question is whether all tumors evoke a response, which may not necessarily be detectable by the methods at present available.

DETECTION AND ASSAY OF TSA AND THEIR ANTIBODIES

The TSA are generally very weak. Antibodies are rarely produced in quantities sufficient for precipitation, although this may occur in special circumstances.[2] The reason why this should be so is clear, at least so far as the surface antigens are concerned. Only those tumors which carry weak antigens can survive and grow; others may occur which carry stronger antigens, but they are presumably eliminated at an early stage and therefore escape detection. This general consideration can be supplemented in several ways. In the case of viral tumors, animals may be infected with endemic viruses of selected type, rendering them immunologically tolerant of shared viral antigens.[3] In at least some cases it is also likely that TSA represent rearrangements of

151

material present near the surface of normal cells, rather than entirely new structures, so that a certain degree of tolerance can again be expected.[4]

This very weakness poses an attractive problem: how can the methods of modern immunology be best applied to the tumor problem? It is this combination of great practical importance with a need for the most sophisticated methods which has stimulated much of the recent interest in cancer immunology. Sooner or later all the new developments in immunology seem to get applied to TSA. Fortunately the subject has been ably reviewed recently on several occasions, notably in three symposia,[5-7] a review[8] and a monograph.[9] Therefore I shall not deal with the subject extensively, but instead offer a classification of methods (Table 1), and a few comments.

Immunization is, in a sense, the method of ultimate reference, because one hopes that sooner or later the TSA will be used for the purpose of clinical immunization. Tests based on immunization have two defects, however, whose importance is illustrated in the recent history of research on transplantation antigens. They are slow and cumbersome. Davies, Nathenson and others who are now sorting out the H-2 and HLA antigens are able to advance so rapidly because in vitro tests are being used. They can also mislead, because for successful immunization not only must the antigen be present, but it must be presented in the right way to elicit cell-mediated immunity. This has caused some misunderstanding over transplantation antigens, where a distinction between "T" antigens (characteristic of tissue cells, and capable of eliciting transplantation immunity) and "H" antigens (characteristic of erythrocytes, and incapable of eliciting transplantation immunity) was at one time proposed. There are no grounds

Table 1.—Methods for Detecting TSA

Methods Based on Immunization
    Increase in resistance/susceptibility to tumor transplantation
        Foley, 1953 [53]
        Prehn and Main, 1957 [1]
        Old, Boyse, Clark and Carswell, 1962 [54]
    Increase in resistance/susceptibility to viral tumor-induction
        Goldner, Girardi, Larson and Hilleman, 1964 [55]
        Rapp, Melnick and Terithia, 1968 [12]
Serological Methods
    Precipitation
        Geering, Old and Boyse, 1966 [2]
        Old, Boyse, Oetgen, de Harven, Geering, Williamson and Clifford, 1966 [56]
    Anti-immunoglobulin sandwich techniques
        Mixed agglutination
            Metzger and Olenick, 1968 [57]
        Fluorescence
            Klein and Klein, 1964 [58]
            Baldwin and Barker, 1967 [59]
        Radioactively-labeled anti-immunoglobulin
            Harder and McKhann, 1968 [60]
        Hybrid antibody
            Hammerling et al. 1968 [61]
        Ferritin-labeled anti-immunoglobulin
            Kalmus, Stitch and Yohn, 1966 [62]
    Complement techniques
        Cytotoxicity
            Klein and Klein, 1964 [58]
        Immune adherence, etc.
            Müller-Eberhard, 1968 [63]
            Nelson, 1968 [64]
    Binding tests
    Labeled ab
        Hammerling (personal communication)
    Labeled ag
Cell-mediated Immunity Methods
    Delayed hypersensitivity in vivo
        Churchill, Rapp, Kronman and Borsos, 1968 [65]
    Inhibition of macrophage migration
        Halliday and Webb, 1969 [66]
    Cytotoxicity
    Hellström, Hellström and Pierce, 1968 [67]

for believing that the determinants on the two cells are different, and instead it seems that antigens on erythrocytes are somehow presented in a manner that fails to elicit cell-mediated immunity.

This has also caused confusion in recent work on the surface antigen of virus-transformed cells. Defendi[10] and Girardi[11] use a test involving inoculation of newborn hamsters with SV_{40} virus followed later by inoculation of cells or cell extracts to reduce tumor incidence. As judged by this test, viable cells, but not killed cells or cell extracts will immunize. On the other hand, Rapp, Melnick and Terithia[12] find that cell extracts are active in immunization against SV_{40} surface antigens. In their test the extracts are inoculated into newborn hamsters, which are thereby rendered susceptible to the later inoculation of live cells transformed by SV_{40} virus. Presumably the second test depends either on induction of tolerance or on enhancement by this extract. Prior experience with transplantation antigens would suggest that enhancement is likely to be less dependent than immunization on the use of viable cells.

The very fact that so many different serological techniques are practiced indicates that no single method has been agreed on as the best. Methods are chosen in order to yield the optimum combination of sensitivity, specificity, and convenience in particular circumstances. The choice depends partly on experience already gained with TSA, and partly on general considerations. Comparisons with studies of antigens located on the surface of cells which participate in the immune response are particularly relevant.

Thus, for example, much effort has been directed toward locating antigen on the surface of macrophages, and particularly antigen on the dendritic processes of the macrophages in lymph node follicles. Antigen was first detected in this location simultaneously and independently by two methods: immunofluorescence and autoradiography. Subsequent careful comparison of the two methods has shown that 100,000 times less antigen (flagellin in the rat) can be detected by autoradiography than by immunofluorescence.[13] Nevertheless, immunofluorescence retains its value as a method that permits topographic localization in detail.

Similarly, the problem of immunoglobulin localization on the lymphocyte surface has attracted attention because of its relevance to antigen recognition in the immune response. Immunoglobulin was first identified in this location by an indirect method, the transformation of lymphocytes by anti-immunoglobulin antibodies.[14] Three of my present colleagues and I have been working on this problem, each of us using anti-immunoglobulin antibodies in different ways. Greaves uses them to opsonise lymphocytes, I use them competitively to inhibit stimulation by antigen, Raff conjugates them with fluorescein and uses them for fluorescence, and Taylor radioiodinates them and makes autoradiographs.[15-17] Meanwhile others are using these antibodies in yet other ways. R. R. A. Coombs, P. G. H. Gell and their colleagues, for example, employ a mixed haemagglutination technique. Not all the results have yet been published, and one confidently expects other work on this problem to appear. Quite apart from their intrinsic importance, all these studies should benefit future work on TSA from a technical point of view. We learn, for example, that when used for autoradiography, antisera can be used at much lower dilutions than when used for immunofluorescence (Raff and Taylor find a difference by a factor of $\times$ 10,000). We suspect that certain methods may yield misleading information with immunoglobulin antisera rendered apparently class specific by absorption, simply on account of their extreme sensitivity which may pick up cross-reactions that escape detection by conventional serological methods. It was surprising to learn that the elegant double-antibody method of Hämmerling has so far not detected immunoglobulin on the surface of lymphocytes (U. Hämmerling, personal communication). Immunologists seem to have laid themselves open to the criticism that they are willing to exert their most sophisticated efforts only for the benefit of their own private problems.

Most serological tests for TSA are, immunologically speaking, "secondary," i.e., they depend on detecting the secondary consequences of the binding of antibody to TSA. As such, they necessarily involve greater complexity and uncertainty than primary reactions, and tend to reveal little about the quality of the antibody. The primary interaction between antigen and antibody is nowadays generally measured by means of radioactive markers on either antigen or antibody. There is a widespread trend toward the use of this kind of test not only because of its more direct character but because tests with radioactive markers are quick, accurate, and easily automated. This applies especially to gamma-emitting isotopes, which can be assayed merely by inserting a test tube into a detector. The Hämmerling method, in which antisera are labelled with tritium, can be regarded as a test of this nature, although it has so far been applied mainly to the reaction between antibody and whole cells. Radioiodination is said to present problems of denaturation with mouse antisera, although we have not encountered such problems in radioiodinating mouse anti-allotype antibody.[18]

The ultimate aim must surely be to measure the interaction between solubilized cell surface antigens and antibody, using a radioactive binding test. Effort is being devoted to working out this method as applied to transplantation antigens in my own laboratory and elsewhere. Once the problem has been cracked for transplantation antigens, the application to TSA will certainly follow.

The drive to develop methods of assessing cellular immunity stems from the belief that only this type of immunity is potentially capable of destroying tumors. Cell-mediated immunity is not a new concept. What is exciting in the new work is that ways have been found of measuring reactivity in vitro, by means of colony inhibition and inhibition of macrophage migration. In addition to all the advantages of any in vitro test, these tests enable us unequivocally to dissect cellular immunity from the inhibitory influence of concomitant humoral immunity ("enhancement").

Nevertheless it would be a pity to forget that promising lines of attack on this problem have also been opened up by recent in vivo cell transfer experiments. Thus, for example, Davies and his colleagues[19] have shown that cells mediating cellular immunity (thymus-derived) can be sorted out from cells mediating antibody production (marrow-derived). Their method depends on the use of marrow/thymus non-H-2 chimaeras, and transfer into appropriately iso-immunized hosts. Another maneuver involves depriving immunized mice of recirculating lymphocytes, which are predominantly thymus-derived and mediators of cellular immunity, by means of ALS, and then restoring humoral reactivity by the transfer of appropriately immunized helper cells. In this way a cell population can be assayed quantitatively for helper activity, which is thought to reflect cellular immunity.[20] Here again one feels that these transplantation methods will find an application in the analysis of the reaction to TSA, even if we have not yet found precisely the right experiment.

COOPERATION BETWEEN LYMPHOCYTES IN INDUCTION OF IMMUNE RESPONSE

Dr. Beverley, Mr. M. Iverson and I have become interested in the possibility of increasing the immune response to TSA by introducing new immunological determinants onto tumor cells, and what follows represents our joint thoughts. The same idea has occurred to several others before and has been implemented in several investigations which follow much the same plan. A new determinant, which may be called the helper determinant, and which can be a hapten, a protein, a viral coat antigen, a transplantation antigen, or a xenogenous cell antigen, is introduced into a population of tumor cells. The cells are then transplanted into an individual who would be expected to tolerate the growth of unmodified tumor cells. Clinically the hope is that the modified cells would be transplanted back into tumor-bearing patients. After transplantation, an immunologic reaction occurs against the helper determinants, as a consequence of which the reaction to the accompanying TSA is increased, and cells which would otherwise be tolerated are destroyed.

One of the first investigations of this nature, and to my mind still the most enterprising and promising, was performed by Lindenmann and Klein.[21] In their study the helper determinant was influenza virus. They found that mice could be immunized against the Ehrlich tumor by inoculation with viral oncolysates of the tumor. When the lysate was fractionated they found that the tumor-immunizing antigen followed the virions. They further found, and this provides the most direct link with subsequent

158

work on thymus-marrow cooperation, that antisera raised against egg-grown virus would specifically inhibit the capacity of oncolysate to immunize against the tumor.

Further work on animal tumors has been at times encouraging[22-26] and at others less so.[27-29] The approach has also been applied to human tumors, again with occasional encouraging results.[30,31] (These references are included in the general collection shown in Table 2.)

The mode of action of the helper determinants is far from clear. One possibility, from an immunological standpoint the most disappointing, is that the helper determinants do not serve an immunologic role at all. The modified cells are merely attenuated, in the sense that their growth rate is slowed down or their susceptibility to immunologic attack increased. This is the argument advanced by Augustin.[28] It applies most strongly to experiments with such tumors as the Ehrlich, with which immunity can in any case be easily obtained. Another possibility, also immunologically fairly trivial, is that the helper determinants merely provide points of attack and so enable the modified cells to be killed by an immune response not directed against TSA. This is the mode of action proposed for the rejection of tumor cells infected with Friend virus.[32,33] One can easily formulate mechanisms intermediate between these two. For example, protection via an immune response against helper determinants might permit relatively large doses of modified tumor cells to be inoculated and a heightened response to TSA thus obtained.

Next there comes a group of possible mechanisms which are immunologically of intermediate interest. Broadly speaking these are when the helper determinants exert an adjuvant action. One possibility is that binding of the helper determinant to

Table 2.—Data Interpretable as Evidence For or Against Cooperation Between
Determinants in Immune Response

Inducing Determinant	Helper Determinant	
Purified Antigens		
Protein	Protein	Rajewsky & Rottländer, 1967 [68]
		Rajewsky, Rottländer, Peltre & Müller, 1967 [69]
		Cohn, Notani & Rice, 1969 [70]
		Taylor, 1969 [48]
		Mitchison, Rajewsky & Taylor, 1969 [52]
		Weigle, 1961 [71]; for discussion of this work see
		Boak, Kölsch & Mitchison, 1969 [72]
Hapten	Protein	Rajewsky, Schirrmacher, Nase & Jerne, 1969 [73]
		Mitchison, 1967 [16]
		Mitchison, 1968 [45]
		Mitchison, 1969 [74]
Protein	Hapten	Mitchison, Rajewsky & Taylor, 1969 [52]
		Mitchison, 1969 [20]
		Leskowitz, 1969 [35]
Polyamino acid	Protein	Green, Paul & Benacerraf, 1966 [75]
Nucleic acid	Protein	Plescia & Braun, 1967 [76]
Protein	Allo	Bloch & Nordin, 1960 [77]; for discussion of this work see
		Mitchison, 1969 [42]

160

Cells		
Tumor	Hapten	Baldwin & Barker, 1967 [27]
Tumor	Allo	Della Porta, Colnaghi & Parmiani, 1969 [23] Skurkovitch, Kisljak, Machonova & Begunenko, 1969 [31]
Tumor	Xeno	Watkins & Chan, 1969 [24] Harris, Miller, Klein, Worst & Tachibana, 1969 [25]
Tumor	Viral	Lindenmann & Klein, 1967 [21] Kobayashi, Sendo, Toshikazu, Hiroshi, Takao & Hiroshi, 1969 [32] Kobayashi, 1969 [33]
Tumor	Protein	Czajkowski, Rosenblatt, Cushing, Vasquez & Wolf, 1966 [22] Czajkowski, Rosenblatt, Wolf & Vasquez, 1967 [30]
Tumor	Protein	Augustin, 1969 [28] Nishioka, Furuse, Inoue, Chang & Takeuchi, 1969 [26] Baldwin & Barker, 1967 [27] McEnany, Kelly & Fahey, 1968 [29]
Auto	Hapten	Weigle, 1965 [78]
Auto	Protein	Weigle, 1961 [71] Chiba, Rosenblatt, Yamanaka, Wolf, Bassenge & Bing, 1965 [79]
Auto	Allo	Favri, 1968 [80]
Allo	Allo	Schierman & McBride, 1967 [36] Schierman, Leckband & McBride, 1969 [37] McBride & Schierman (personal communication) Cantor, H.I. & Asofski, R. (personal communication) Berrian & McKhann, 1960 [34]
Xeno	Xeno	Davies, Leuchars, Wallis, Marchant & Elliott, 1967 [19] Miller & Mitchell, 1969 [47]

antibody, perhaps in a cell-bound form, results in a steric interaction which increases the immunogenic activity of adjacent TSA. Another possibility, suggested by Berrian and McKhan,[34] who very kindly attribute the idea to me, is that the response to the helper determinant promotes localization of the cells in the right part of the body for immunization, in particular in lymph nodes. A third possibility suggested by Leskowitz[35] is pharmacologic in nature. Helper determinants that induce a delayed-hypersensitivity response thereby liberate chemical mediators, and these attract host cells such as macrophages. This, in turn, provides a cellular environment that encourages the response to the accompanying determinants.

There is also a group of possible mechanisms in which the helper determinants play a very particular role. These have been the subject of a great deal of recent work, most of which has nothing ostensibly to do with tumors but which is nevertheless highly relevant (see Table 2). This work has been carried out in three kinds of system. One system involves enhancing the response to antigens, usually erythrocytes, by means of soluble antibody. McBride and Schierman have shown that the response to the weak A-isoantigens in chickens can be enhanced by a concomitant response to the strong B-isoantigens[36,37] and have gone on to examine the mechanism of enhancement in detail. For enhancement to be obtained, the two isoantigens must be presented on the same erythrocyte. The enhancement can itself be increased by passive antibody to the helper isoantigens or by immunizing with erythrocytes precoated with anti-helper antibody. Steric or gross localization effects of the kind mentioned above can be largely excluded, for precoating only works if the recipient is incompatible for the precoated determinant. Allied experiments have been

162

performed by Henry and Jerne[38] on the response of mice to sheep erythrocytes. They find that this response can be enhanced by 19S antibody to the erythrocytes but not by 7S antibody. Another example of the remarkable in vivo activity of this type of antibody can be found in the work of Rowley, Turner and Jenkins[39] who were able to show that the capacity to transfer immunity to mouse typhoid adoptively by peritoneal macrophages is due to cell-bound antibody. This antibody, which could be eluted with 2M urea, is also a macroglobulin. It appears to share properties in common with the cell-supernatants which are being found to have helper activity in the sheep red cell response.[40]

The interrelationship between these soluble factors is not yet clear, nor do we know whether any of them may be IgX, the hypothetical thymus-derived · antibody.[41] Provisionally perhaps it is best to put them in a category of their own, separate from the cell-mediated, thymus-dependent helper effects that are to be described below. If this distinction is valid and both are fundamentally antigen-concentrating mechanisms as has been suggested,[42,43] we should expect them to act non-synergistically. Antibody-mediated helper effects should be most generally demonstrable and most powerful when cell-mediated effects are not operating, e.g., after thymectomy. The same applies to macrophage-mediated helper effects if these are also a matter of antigen concentration.[44,45] According to this view, a weak antigen needs whatever help it can get in presentation to receptors on antibody-forming-cell-precursors. If one mechanism is not operating then others become all the more vital.

The second helper system which has received much recent attention is cooperation between thymus-derived and marrow-derived lymphocytes. The generally accepted view at present is that antibody-forming cells are descended from lymphocytes which have not passed through the thymus, and which are potentially capable of recognising and reacting to antigens. Nevertheless, this reaction cannot always take place without the help of specifically reactive, thymus-derived cells. The thymus-derived cells are thought to pick up the antigen by one determinant and present it to the thymus-independent cell, which is then able to react against other determinants.[46-49]

The third helper system which has recently been clarified is the role of the carrier in the response to haptens conjugated to proteins. It has long been known that an individual immunized with a hapten on carrier protein A will fail to make a secondary response to the same hapten on carrier protein B, and similar rules apply to delayed hypersensitivity and to immunologic tolerance.[50] It is now thought that a major part of these carrier effects can be accounted for by anti-carrier antibody exerting a helper effect,[51,52] and it is strongly suspected that the carrier antibody is carried on thymus-derived cells which carry it in cell-bound form. If this view is correct the carrier effect is identical with the thymus-marrow interaction referred to above. Other consequences also follow. This form of helper effect could then be distinguished, as was suggested above, from helper effects mediated by secreted antibody, and the appropriate strategy for activating them in respect of TSA will involve stimulation of cellular immunity. The precise role of cellular immunity therefore becomes a matter of importance, and it is worth listing the evidence in support (details in references cited above and in Table 2; for theta from M. Raff, unpublished data; and for thoracic duct cells from J. L. Boak, A. Pattisson and N. A.

Mitchison, unpublished data).

(1) Helper effects have not been obtained with passively transferred anti-carrier antibody.

(2) Helper activity appears relatively soon after immunization, compared with humoral antibody, and therefore displays the characteristic tempo of cellular immunity.

(3) Helper activity, in cell transfer experiments, is highly susceptible to anti-Θ-antibody (applied in vitro) and to anti-lymphocyte serum (applied in vivo). Both agents act differentially on the thymus-derived, recirculating lymphocytes which are thought to be responsible for cell-mediated immunity.

(4) Skin-painting with reactive haptens, a traditional method of evoking cell-mediated immunity, elicits helper cells but little humoral antibody (in these experiments the helper reactivity is directed towards the dinitrophenyl hapten used and not toward the carrier).

(5) Thoracic duct lymphocytes as compared with spleen cells are relatively richer in helper cells than in antibody-forming cell precursors. Lymphocytes from the thoracic duct belong largely to the recirculating pool.

(6) "Activated" thymus-derived cells, obtained from lethally-irradiated, thymocyte-repopulated, immunized donors are high in helper activity.

Two further points are particularly relevant to future experiments with TSA. First, the distinction between hapten and carrier is only relative. The traditional haptens, such as the dinitrophenyl group, can subserve a helper function, and there is no theoretical reason why they should not be used on cells. While there is no direct evidence that helper activity can increase a cell-mediated response, the indirect evidence of carrier effects in delayed hyper-sensitivity suggests that this should be possible. This is reassuring, because obviously we do not want to use maneuvers which will increase only the level of enhancing antibodies.

What moral then should we draw from this survey of what has so far been found out? It seems to me that we cannot yet make a final judgment. On one hand we have a detailed body of information about the working of cooperation in certain well-defined systems that lend themselves to laboratory study, and on the other we have a long and not entirely encouraging history of effort at exploiting cooperation for tumor immunotherapy. Certainly no one has yet settled down to a program of evaluating all the possibilities that are on offer for this purpose. The collection of helper determinants listed in Table 2 deserve systematic study. Haptens, for example, have the advantages of being well-defined, easily quantitated, and well adapted for raising cell-mediated immunity. Viruses, naturally-occurring surface antigens, and antigens induced by hybridization have the contrasting advantage of being propagated as cells multiply, and then there are all the questions concerning the possible advantages of prior or concomitant sensitization against the helper determinants that need to be answered. I foresee an interesting body of research to come.

REFERENCES

1. Prehn, R. T., and Main, J. M.: Immunity to methylcholanthrene-induced sarcomas. J. Nat. Cancer Inst. 18:769, 1957.

2. Geering, G., Old, L. J., and Boyse, E. A.: Antigens of leukemias induced by naturally-occurring murine leukemia virus: Their relation to the antigens of Gross virus and other murine leukemia viruses. J. Exp. Med. 124:753, 1966.

3. Old, L. J., Boyse, E. A., Geering, G., and Oettgen, H. F.: Serological approaches to the

study of cancer in animals and in man. Cancer Res. 28:1288, 1968.

4. Burger, M. M.: A difference in the architecture of the surface membrane of normal and virally transformed cells. Proc. Nat. Acad. Sci. 62: 994, 1969.

5. Symposium on Immunopathology of Cancer. Fed. Proc. 24:1007, 1965.

6. Symposium on Tumor-specific antigens. Cancer Res. 28:1275, 1969.

7. Conference on Viral, tumor, and transplantation antigen isolation, Oak Ridge, Tenn. Transplantation 6:632, 1968.

8. Smith, R. T.: Tumor-specific immune mechanism. New Eng. J. Med. 278:1207, 1268, 1968.

9. Koldovsky, P.: Tumor specific transplantation antigen. Recent Results in Cancer Research. New York, Springer-Verlag New York, 1969.

10. Defendi, V.: Studies with virally-induced transplantation antigens. Transplantation 6:642, 1968.

11. Girardi, A. J.: Studies of prevention of SV_{40}-induced tumors in hamsters. Transplantation 6:643, 1968.

12. Rapp, F., Melnick, J. L., and Terithia, S. S.: Genetic factors governing the control of virus-induced tumor, surface and transplantation antigens and immunologic characterization of those antigens. Transplantation 6:649, 1968.

13. Miller, J. J., and Nossal, G. J. V.: Antigens in immunity. VI. The phagocytic reticulum of lymph node follicles. J. Exp. Med. 120:1075, 1964.

14. Sell, S., and Gell, P. G. H.: Studies on rabbit lymphocytes in vitro. I. Stimulation of blast transformation with an antiallotype serum. J. Exp. Med. 122:423, 1965.

15. Greaves, M., and Roitt, I.: Personal communication.

16. Mitchison, N. A.: Antigen recognition responsible for the induction in vitro of the secondary response. Cold Spr. Harb. Symp. Quant. Biol. 32:431, 1967.

17. Raff, M., Sternberg, M., and Taylor, R. B.: Immunoglobulin determinants on the surface of mouse lymphoid cells. Nature (London) (in press).

18. Bomford, R., Breitner, J., Mitchison, N. A., Negroni, N., and Raff, M.: Detection of cellular antigens by cytotoxicity, radio-uptake and other methods. Paper presented at the International Conference on "Immunity and Tolerance in Oncogenesis, Perugia, Italy, 1969.

167

19. Davies, A. J. S., Leuchars, E., Wallis, V., Marchant, R., and Elliott, E. V.: The failure of thymus-derived cells to produce antibody. Transplantation 5:222, 1967.

20. Mitchison, N. A.: Mechanism of action of antilymphocyte serum. Fed. Proc. (in press).

21. Lindenmann, J., and Klein, P. A.: Viral oncolysis: increased immunogenicity of host cell antigen associated with influenza virus. J. Exp. Med. 126:93, 1967.

22. Czajkowski, N. P., Rosenblatt, M., Cushing, F. R., Vasquez, J., and Wolf, P. L.: Production of active immunity to active neoplastic tissue: Chemical coupling to an antigenic protein carrier. Cancer 19:739, 1966.

23. Della Porta, G., Colnaghi, M. I., and Parmiani, G.: Immunological studies of chemically-induced murine lymphosarcomas. Paper presented at the International Conference on Immunity and Tolerance in Oncogenesis, Perugia, Italy, 1969.

24. Watkins, J. F., and Chan, L.: Immunization of mice against Ehrlich ascites tumour using a Hamster/Ehrlich Ascites tumour hybrid cell line. Nature (London) 223:1018, 1969.

25. Harris, H., Miller, O. J., Klein, M., Worst, P., and Tachibana, T.: Suppression of malignancy by cell fusion. Nature (London) 223:363, 1969.

26. Nishioka, K., Furuse Irie, R., Inoue, M., Chang, S., and Takeuchi, S.: Immunological studies on mouse mammary tumors. I. Induction of resistance to tumor isograft in C3H/He mice. Int. J. Cancer 4:121, 1969.

27. Baldwin, R. W., and Barker, C. R.: Immunization against human tumours. Lancet 2: 1090, 1967.

28. Augustin, R.: Immunity against cancer. Nature (London) 224:295, 1969.

29. McEnany, M. T., Kelly, M. G., and Fahey, J. L.: Effects of immunization with tumor-cell-foreign-protein conjugates on growth of syngeneic tumor grafts. Amer. Ass. Cancer Res. 9:46, 1968.

30. Czajkowski, N. P., Rosenblatt, M., Wolf, P. L., and Vasquez, J.: A new method of active immunisation to autologous tumour tissue. Lancet 2:905, 1967.

31. Skurkovitch, S. V., Kisljak, N. S., Machonova, L. A., and Begunenko, S. A.: Active immunisation of children suffering from acute phase with "live" allogeneic leukaemia cells. Nature (London) 223: 509, 1969.

32. Kobayashi, H., Sendo, F., Toshikazu, S., Hiroshi, K., Takao, K., and Hiroshi, S.: Modifica-

tion in growth of transplantable rat tumours exposed to Friend virus. J. Nat. Cancer Inst. 42: 413, 1969.

33. Kobayashi, H.: Modification in growth of rat tumors exposed to Friend virus. Paper presented at the International Conference on Immunity and Tolerance in Oncogenesis, Perugia, Italy, 1969.

34. Berrian, J. H., and McKhann, C. F.: Strength of histocompatibility genes. Ann. N. Y. Acad. Sci. 87:106, 1960.

35. Leskowitz, S.: Is delayed sensitivity a preparation for antibody synthesis? Paper presented at the symposium on Developmental Aspects of Antibody Formation and Structure, Prague, 1969.

36. Schierman, L. W., and McBride, R. A.: Adjuvant activity of erythrocyte isoantigens. Science 156:658, 1967.

37. —, Leckband, E., and McBride, R. A.: Immunological interaction of erythrocyte isoantigens: Effects of passive antibody. Proc. Soc. Exp. Biol. Med., N. Y. 130:744, 1969.

38. Henry, C., and Jerne, N. K.: The depressive effect of 7S antibody and the enhancing effect of 19S antibody in the regulation of the primary immune response. In Killander, J. (Ed.): Nobel Symposium No. 3: Gamma Globulins. New York, Interscience, 1967, p. 431.

39. Rowley, D., Turner, K. J., and Jenkins, C. R.: The basis for immunity to mouse typhoid. III. Cell-bound antibody. Austr. J. Exp. Biol. Med. Sci. 42:237, 1964.

40. Dutton, R.: Paper presented at the conference on Antilymphocyte Serum, Brook Lodge, 1969.

41. Dupuy, J.-M., Perey, D. Y. E., and Good, R. A.: Passive transfer, with plasma, of delayed allergy in guinea pigs. Lancet 1:551, 1969.

42. Mitchison, N. A.: Paper presented at the symposium on Mediators of Cellular Immunity, Brook Lodge, 1969.

43. —: Cellular and molecular recognition mechanisms prior to the immune response. In: Handbuch der Allgemeinen Pathologie. Berlin, Springer-Verlag, 1969.

44. Unanue, E. R., and Askonas, B. A.: Two functions of macrophages and their role in the immune response. J. Reticulo-endothelial Soc. 4: 440, 1967.

45. Mitchison, N. A.: Recognition of antigen. In Warren, K. B. (Ed.): Differentiation and Immunology, Vol. 7. New York, Academic, 1968.

46. Claman, H. N., and Chaperon, E. A.: Im-

munological complementation between thymus and marrow cells: A model for the two-cell theory of immunocompetence. Transplantation Rev. 1:92, 1969.

47. Miller, J. F. A. P., and Mitchell, G. F.: Thymus and antigen-reactive cells. Transplantation Rev. 1:3, 1969.

48. Taylor, R. B.: Cellular cooperation in the antibody response of mice to two serum albumins: Specific function of thymus cells. Transplantation Rev. 1:114, 1969.

49. Davies, A. J. S.: The thymus and the cellular basis of immunity. Transplantation Rev. 1:43, 1969.

50. Mitchison, N. A.: Recognition of antigen by cells. In Butler, J. A. V., and Huxley, H. E. (Eds.): Progress in Biophysics, Vol. 16. Oxford, Pergamon, 1966, p. 3.

51. Bretscher, P. A., and Cohn, M.: Minimal model for the mechanism of antibody induction and paralysis by antigen. Nature (London) 220: 444, 1968.

52. Mitchison, N. A., Rajewsky, K., and Taylor, R. B.: Cooperation of antigenic determinants and of cells in the induction of antibodies. Paper presented at the symposium on Developmental Aspects of Antibody Formation and Structure, Prague, 1969.

53. Foley, E. J.: Antigenic properties of methyl-cholanthrene-induced tumors in mice of the strain of origin. Cancer Res. 13:835, 1953.

54. Old, L. J., Boyse, E. A., Clark, D. A., and Carswell, E. A.: Antigenic properties of chemically-induced tumors. Ann. N. Y. Acad. Sci. 101:80, 1962.

55. Goldner, H., Girardi, A. J., Larson, V. M., and Hilleman, M. R.: Interruption of SV_{40} virus tumorigenesis using irradiated homologous tumor antigen. Proc. Soc. Exp. Biol. 117:851, 1964.

56. Old, L. J., Boyse, E. A., Oetgen, H. F., deHarven, E., Geering, G., Williamson, B., and Clifford, P.: Precipitating antibody in human serum to an antigen present in cultured Burkitt's lymphoma cells. Proc. Nat. Acad. Sci. 56:1699, 1966.

57. Metzger, R. S., and Olenick, S. R.: The study of normal and malignant cell antigens by mixed agglutination. Cancer Res. 28:1366, 1968.

58. Klein, G., and Klein, E.: Antigenic properties of lymphomas induced by the Moloney agent. J. Nat. Cancer Inst. 32:547, 1964.

59. Baldwin, R. W., and Barker, C. R.: Demon-

170

stration of tumor-specific humoral antibody against amino-azo dye-induced rat hepatoma. Brit. J. Cancer 21:793, 1967.

60. Harder, F. H., and McKhann, C. F.: Demonstration of cellular antigens on sarcoma cells by an indirect ^{125}I-labelled antibody technique. J. Nat. Cancer Inst. 40:231, 1968.

61. Hämmerling, U., Aoki, T., deHarven, E., Boyse, E. A., and Old, L. J.: Use of hybrid antibody with anti-Ig and anti-ferritin specificities in locating cell surface antigens by electron microscopy. J. Exp. Med. 128:1461, 1968.

62. Kalmus, V. I., Stitch, H. F., and Yohn, D. S.: Electron microscopic localisation of virus-associated antigens in human amnion cells (AV-3) infected with human adeno-virus. Virology 28:751, 1966.

63. Müller-Eberhard, H. J.: The possible use of complement for the detection of cell surface antigens. Cancer Res. 28:1357, 1968.

64. Nelson, R. A.: The role of cellular antigens in complement-induced cytocidal, immune adherence, and phagocytic reactions. Cancer Res. 28: 1361, 1968.

65. Churchill, W. H., Jr., Rapp, H. J., Kronman, B. S., and Borsos, T.: Detection of antigens of a new diethylnitrosamine-induced transplantable hepatoma by delayed hypersensitivity. J. Nat. Cancer Inst. 41:13, 1968.

66. Halliday, W. J., and Webb, M.: Delayed hypersensitivity to chemically-induced tumors in mice and correlation with an in vitro test. J. Nat. Cancer Inst. 43:141, 1969.

67. Hellström, I., Hellström, K. E., and Pierce, G. E.: In vitro studies of immune reactions against autochthonous and syngeneic mouse tumours induced by methylcholanthrene and plastic discs. Int. J. Cancer 3:467, 1968.

68. Rajewsky, K., and Rottländer, E.: Tolerance specificity and the immune response to lactic dehydrogenase isoenzymes. Cold. Spr. Harb. Symp. Quant. Biol. 32:547, 1967.

69. Rajewsky, K., Rottländer, E., Peltre, G., and Müller, B.: The immune response to a hybrid protein molecule. Specificity of secondary stimulation and tolerance induction. J. Exp. Med. 126: 581, 1967.

70. Cohn, M., Notani, G., and Rice, S. A.: Characterisation of the antibody to the C-carbohydrate produced by a transplantable mouse plasmacytoma. Immunochemistry 6:111, 1969.

71. Weigle, W. O.: The immune response of

171

rabbits tolerant to BSA to the injection of other
heterologous serum albumins. J. Exp. Med. 114:
111, 1961.

72. Boak, J. L., Kölsch, E., and Mitchison,
N. A.: Immunological tolerance and inhibition by
hapten. Antibiot. Chemother. (Basel) 15:98, 1969.

73. Rajewsky, K., Schirrmacher, V., Nase, S.,
and Jerne, N. K.: The requirement of more than
one antigenic determinant for immunogenicity. J.
Exp. Med. 129:1131, 1969.

74. Mitchison, N. A.: Transplantation immunology. In: Organ Transplantation Today. New
York, Excerpta Medica Foundation, 1969, p. 13.

75. Green, I., Paul, W. E., and Benacerraf, B.:
The behaviour of hapten-poly-L-lysine conjugates
as complete antigens in genetic responders and as
haptens in non-responder guinea-pigs. J. Exp.
Med. 123:859, 1966.

76. Plescia, O. J., and Braun, W.: Nucleic
acids as antigens. Adv. Immunol. 6:231, 1967.

77. Bloch, H., and Nordin, A. A.: Production
of tuberculin sensitivity. Nature (London) 187:
434, 1960.

78. Weigle, W. O.: The induction of auto-
immunity in rabbits following injection of heterologous or altered homologous thyroglobulin. J.
Exp. Med. 121:289, 1965.

79. Chiba, C., Rosenblatt, M., Yamanaka, J.,
Wolf, P. L., Bassenge, E., and Bing, R. J.: Im-
munologically produced lymphopenia. Arch. Int.
Med. 115:558, 1965.

80. Fravi, G.: Präzipitierende Leber-Auto-
antikörper bei der Maus. Path. Microbiol. (Basel)
31:257, 1968.

TREATMENT OF CHRONIC MUCOCUTANEOUS
MONILIASIS BY IMMUNOLOGIC RECONSTITUTION

C. H. KIRKPATRICK, R. R. RICH, R. G. GRAW, Jr, T. K. SMITH, IRAD,
MICKENBERG AND G. N. ROGENTINE

SUMMARY

The immunological defect in a patient with chronic mucocutaneous moniliasis was characterized. While his Candida skin test was negative. exposure of his lymphocytes to candida extracts *in vitro* produced an increase in thymidine incorporation. Supernatants from cultures of antigen-stimulated lymphocytes did not contain macrophage migration-inhibition factor (MIF) activity.

Restoration of the immune system with transfusions of immuno-competent allogeneic lymphocytes was accompanied by conversion of the Candida skin test to positive, and MIF production by his lymphocytes. During the period that his immune system remained intact, there was marked clearing of the moniliasis. Eight months following the transfusions, the moniliasis recurred and when restudied, the patient again had negative skin tests and insignificant MIF production.

These observations demonstrate the importance of mediators in the expression of delayed hypersensitivity and provide evidence of a role of cellular immunity in resistance to certain chronic fungal infections.

INTRODUCTION

The role of immunologic factors in resistance to infection with *Candida albicans* is poorly understood, however, several observations have indicated the importance of the cellular immune system. Infants with congenital absence or dysplasia of the thymus have a high incidence of moniliasis (Hermans, Ulrich & Markowitz, 1969), and in one instance, restoration of immune competence with a thymus transplant, was accompanied by clearing of the monilia infection (Cleveland *et al.*, 1968).

Recently it has been shown that lymphocytes from animals or human subjects with delayed hypersensitivity respond to antigenic stimulation *in vitro* by replicating (Ling, 1968) and producing substances with diverse biological activities such as chemotaxis (Ward, Rémold & David 1969), cytotoxicity (Granger & Williams, 1968), inhibition of migration of macrophages (David, 1968) and non-specific recruitment of lymphocytes into DNA synthesis (Maini *et al.*, 1968; Kirkpatrick *et al.*, 1970). These substances are presumed to be 'mediators' involved in the pathogenesis of lesions of cellular hypersensitivity.

This report describes a patient with chronic mucocutaneous moniliasis and hypoparathyroidism in whom a defect in the cellular immune system was characterized. Because amphotericin-B induced remissions in these patients are rarely sustained, it was elected to attempt immunologic reconstitution. Transfusion of immuno-competent lymphocytes temporarily corrected the defect and was accompanied by marked clearing of the moniliasis.

CASE REPORT

The patient, a 17-year-old Caucasian male, was admitted to the National Institute of Allergy and Infectious Diseases in May 1969, for investigation of chronic mucocutaneous moniliasis. He developed severe 'diaper rash' at 6 months. *Candida albicans* was cultured from the eruption. The skin lesions progressed and by 18 months of age involved the scalp, face, ears, neck, back and distal extremities, as well as the nails and buccal cavity. At age 7 years the serum calcium and phosphorus levels were 10·5 and 4·5 mg per 100 ml respectively. At a routine examination 5 years later, the serum calcium and phosphorus concentrations were 6·5 and 9·4 mg per 100 ml although the patient had no symptoms of hypocalcemia. He was referred to the National Heart Institute where the diagnosis of primary hypoparathyroidism was established. Although there have been periods of drug resistance, in general the response to treatment with calcium gluconate, dihydrotachysterol or 25-hydroxycholecalciferol has been satisfactory.

Severe dysplasia of the dental enamel led to complete extractions in 1964. The extent and severity of the moniliasis have varied through the years, but the general course had been one of progression. There had been no sustained response to nystatin, gentian violet or topical amphotericin-B. With the exception of numerous hospitalizations for evaluation and treatment of moniliasis and an episode of pneumococcal septicemia at age 18 months, the past history was unremarkable. The patient had no unusual incidence of viral infections, and there were no known allergies.

Upon admission to the National Institute of Allergy and Infectious Diseases, the general physical examination revealed numerous erythematous, firm, elevated, crusting lesions over the scalp, neck (Fig. la), back, groin, and distal extremities (Figs 2a, 3a, 4a), and extensive destruction of the nails (Fig. 5). The external auditory canals were scaly and contained serous exudates. Both tympanic membranes were thickened and the right membrane had a large perforation. The mouth was edentulous and many large patches of thrush were present over the membranes of the tongue and buccal cavity. Several 1–2 cm firm, non-tender lymph nodes were felt in the cervical and supraclavicular areas, and the spleen tip was 2–3 cm below the left costal margin. Chvostek's sign was positive.

No other members of the family were known to have endocrinopathies immunological abnormalities or moniliasis, and there was no history of consanquinity.

Routine laboratory studies such as the peripheral blood count, urinalysis, blood urea nitrogen, creatinine, fasting and post-prandial glucose, electrolytes and liver function tests were normal. The serum calcium varied between 7·2 and 8·8 and the phosphorus between 5·0 and 5·9 mg per 100 ml. The serum iron was 65 μg per 100 ml. Studies of endocrine

174

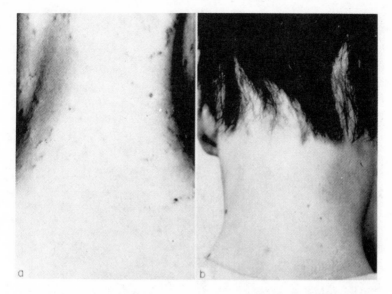

FIG. 1. (a) Cutaneous moniliasis involving the skin of the neck (May, 1969). (b) Marked clearing of the lesions occurred three weeks following the lymphocyte transfusions. There was also marked improvement of the alopecia.

gland and gastrointestinal functions are summarized in Table 1. Cultures of the buccal cavity, skin, scalp, and nails yielded *Candida albicans*, Group A, but there was no growth from the urine, blood or bone marrow.

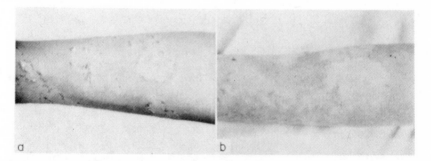

FIG. 2. (a) Cutaneous moniliasis of the skin of the forearm (May, 1969). (b) Same area three weeks after leucocyte transfusions. There was marked loss of the erythematous plaques with temporary depigmentation of the healed areas.

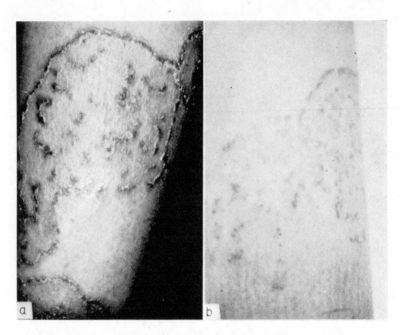

FIG. 3. (a) Moniliasis involving skin of the calf (May, 1969). (b) Three weeks after the leucocyte transfusions there was marked improvement in the cutaneous lesions. Only soft erythema remains.

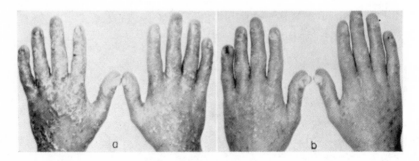

FIG. 4. (a) Moniliasis of the hands and nails (May, 1969). (b) Partial clearing of the cutaneous lesions 5 weeks following the leucocyte transfusions. There was essentially no change in the nails.

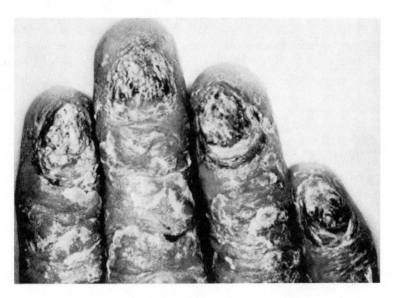

Fɪɢ. 5. (a) Chronic moniliasis involving the nails of skin of fingers.

Tᴀʙʟᴇ 1. Endocrinological and gastrointestinal function studies

Serum calcium		7·30–8·80 mg/100 ml
Serum phosphorus		5·0–5·9 mg/100 ml
Parathormone test	Baseline	After 1500 units PTH
Serum Ca (mg/100 ml)	6·30–8·40	12·8
Serum P (mg/100 ml)	9·0 –9·6	4·9
ACTH Test	Baseline	Max. excretion after stimulation
17-OH Steroids (mg/24 hr urine)	5·6	21·8
17-Ketogenic Steroids (mg/25 hr urine)	4·3	4·3
PBI (μg per 100 ml)	5·6 (Normal 4·0–8·0)	
T₄ (column) (μg per 100 ml)	5·0 (Normal 3·1–6·7)	
T₃ (per cent)	32·5 (Normal 25–35)	

Serum Carotene (units) 142 (normal 100–300)
D-xylose-1·8 g excreted in 5 hr after 5 g oral dose
Gastric acidity–Positive by Diagnex blue test

177

Intradermal skin tests. Cutaneous responses of the patient and his father were studied with a panel of commercial antigens including intermediate and second strength PPD, histoplasmin, mumps, streptokinase-streptodornase (SK-SD, Varidase, Lederle Laboratories, Pearl River, New York) diluted to contain 400 units and 100 units or 40 units and 10 units per 0·1 ml, and dermatophytin (Hollister-Stier Laboratories, Downers Grove, Ill.) 1:100. An additional antigenic extract was prepared by sonically disrupting *C. albicans* isolated from the patient (Kirkpatrick, Chandler and Schimke, 1970). This material was standardized by determining the minimal dose producing 0·5 cm of induration at 24 or 48 hr following intradermal inoculation into healthy subjects known to have delayed allergy to *C. albicans*. Repeated intradermal tests applied to subjects with negative skin tests, demonstrated that the test antigen was not sensitizing in the dosages employed.

All antigens were injected in a volume of 0·1 ml and the cutaneous sites were examined at 15 min for immediate wheal and flare responses, 6–8 hr for Arthus-like reactions and 24 and 48 hr for delayed hypersensitivity. Delayed reactions with 0·5 cm of induration were considered positive.

Two thousand micrograms of 1-chloro 2,4-dinitrobenzene (CDNB) in acetone were applied to the medial aspect of the upper arm to induce contact allergy. Two weeks later the subjects were challenged by application of 50 μg and 100 μg of the substance of the flexor surface of the forearm.

In vitro studies of lymphocyte functions. The technique for measuring antigen-induced thymidine incorporation in short duration lymphocyte cultures differed slightly from that described previously (Newberry *et al.*, 1968). The tubes contained $2·0 \times 10^6$ lymphocytes in a volume of 2·0 ml of Eagle's minimal essential medium with 15% autologous or homologous plasma, and the cells were exposed to tritiated thymidine during the final four hours of culture.

Macrophage migration inhibition factor (MIF) production in antigen-stimulated and control lymphocyte cultures was measured by methods similar to those described by Thor *et al.* (1968) and Rocklin, Meyers & David (1970). Ten micrograms of the soluble candida sonicate (Kirkpatrick, Chandler & Schimke, 1970) were added to the antigen-stimulated cultures at the beginning of the culture period and after each medium change. The media were collected daily for three days and pooled supernatants were concentrated five-fold by ultrafiltration. Control fluids containing tissue culture media from unstimulated cells or tissue culture media containing no cells, but the same amount of antigen were also prepared and concentrated in the same manner. The supernatants were then added to three Sykes-Moore chambers (Bellco Glass Co., Vineland, N.J.), each containing two capillary tubes filled with guinea-pig peritoneal macrophages. The areas of migration were measured at 16 hr and MIF activity was calculated by the method of Thor *et al.* (1968). Reduction of the area of migration by 20% or more was significant ($P < 0·02$).

Mixed lymphocyte cultures were performed using the 'one-way' method of Bach & Voynow (1966). The cells were labelled with tritiated thymidine during the last 4 hr, and the cultures were harvested on the seventh day.

Serological studies. Candida agglutinins in serum and parotid fluid were measured as described elsewhere (Kirkpatrick *et al.*, 1970) and precipitins were detected by double diffusion in agar gel (Ouchterlony, 1962).

The concentration of IgG, IgA and IgM in the serum was determined by radial diffusion (Mancini, Carbonara & Heremans, 1965) using commercial antibody containing agar gels (Hyland Laboratories, Los Angeles, Calif.). Rheumatoid factor, anti-nuclear antibodies, antithyroglobulin, and the lupus erythematosus factor were assayed by standard laboratory methods. Antibodies against gastric parietal cells, thyroid and adrenal tissues were measured in the laboratory of Dr Robert Blizzard.

Phagocytosis and metabolic properties of leucocytes. The capacity of the patient's and normal leucocytes to ingest and kill micro-organisms was studied with *S. albus*, and *C. albicans* (Mickenberg, Root & Wolff, 1970). Oxidative reactions of leucocytes subsequent to phagocytosis were studied in phagocytic mixtures as previously described (Mickenberg *et al.*, 1970).

Histology of inflammatory exudates. Migration of leucocytes into an area of cutaneous abrasion was studied as described by Rebuck & Crowley (1955).

Leucocyte and erythrocyte typing. Lymphocytes from the patient and members of his family were tested for HL-A antigens by the microcytotoxicity method of Mittal *et al.* (1968), and the HL-A genotypes were determined. Donor and recipient sera were also screened for preformed cytotoxic antibodies by the same technique.

Erythrocyte phenotypes were determined in the Clinical Center Blood Bank by standard methods.

Leucocyte transfusions. Leucocytes were collected from the patient's father using the NCI-IBM continuous flow blood cell separator (Buchner *et al.*, 1969). Four leucophoresis were performed in 5 days during which $92 \cdot 2 \times 10^9$ leucocytes containing $63 \cdot 6 \times 10^9$ lymphocytes were collected. The cells were collected in plastic bags (Transfer Pack, Fenwal Laboratories, Norton Grove, Ill.), containing acid-citrate-dextrose (ACD, NIH formula A) and were transfused into the recipient within 1 hr of collection.

RESULTS

Cutaneous hypersensitivity. The patient developed no immediate or delayed cutaneous reactions to intermediate or second strength tuberculin, histoplasmin, streptokinase-streptodornase or Hollister-Stier dermatophytin, but 0·6 cm of erythema and soft induration appeared at the site of the mumps skin test (Table 2). Fifteen minutes after injection of 1·0 μg of the Candida sonicate, a 2·0 cm pruritic wheal and flare response occurred which subsided in 30 min. At 6 hr the injection site became somewhat indurated, tender and erythematous, but never haemorrhagic or necrotic. This response also subsided, and at 24 hr there was no residual erythema or induration. Subsequent studies with the same antigen in doses containing 0·1 to 100 μg of protein also failed to produce a delayed cutaneous response.

No vesiculation occurred at the site of application of the sensitizing dose of CDNB, and topical challenges with 50 and 100 μg 14 and 38 days later were negative.

The patient's father developed significant reactions to mumps, SK-SD and *C. albicans* and sensitization with 2000 μg of CDNB produced strong contact allergy.

From Table 2 it is apparent that passive transfer of delayed cutaneous responses to SK-SD, *C. albicans* and CDNB accompanied the leucocyte transfusions. Cutaneous responses to CDNB were still present at 14 days, but at 37 days only erythema was observed and subsequent tests were entirely negative. The cutaneous responses to SK-SD and

C. albicans remained positive for 190 days, but both had reverted to negative when he was re-studied at 315 days. Interpretation of the mumps skin test prior to transfusion was difficult because of the absence of definite induration. However, following the leucocyte transfusions well demarcated induration was found. This response also reverted to the previous soft induration at 315 days.

Lymphocyte transformation. In vitro stimulation of the patient's lymphocytes with the candida extract produced an increase in thymidine incorporation (Table 3). Peak responses occurred in cultures stimulated with 5·0 μg of antigen protein per ml, but other doses also

TABLE 2. Delayed cutaneous hypersensitivity response of the patient and his father before and after leucocyte transfusions

Antigen	Recipient Pre-transfusion	Donor (Father)	Recipient Post-transfusion (days)							
			1	7	14	24	37	149	190	315
Mumps	0·6*	1·8	0·5	0·3	1·5	1·5	0·9	0·7	0·7	0·6
C. albicans										
Hollister-Stier 1:100	0	0	0	0	0·5	0	0·7	0·9	0·5	0
Autologous *C. albicans*										
100 μg	0	—	—	—	—	—	—	—	—	0
10 μg	0	2·0	0·2	0·9	1·0	1·2	1·7	0·9	1·1	0
1 μg	0	0·4	0	0	0	0	0·5	0·7	1·0	0
SK-SD										
4000/1000 units	0	—	—	—	1·2	1·4	1·0	0·9	0·8	0
400/100 units	0	9·0	0·5	0·7	0	1·9	0·5	—	—	0
CDNB										
100 μg	0	+	+		+		eryth 0		0	
PPD	0	0	0		—		0		0	
Histoplasmin	0	0	0		—		0		0	

* cm induration at 24 hr.

provided some stimulation. Although the amplitude of the thymidine response was somewhat lower than control subjects, peak responses with the patient's cells occurred at the same dose. Mumps skin test antigen that had been dialyzed free of merthiolate, and phytohaemagglutinin-M also stimulated thymidine incorporation by the patient's lymphocytes. No significant changes in the thymidine response were noted when the patient's cells were cultured in homologous rather than autologous plasma, and the patient's plasma had no effect on the responses of cells from skin test positive donors. Although not shown on the table, subjects with negative skin tests had a two-fold or less increase in thymidine incorporation when their lymphocytes were stimulated with *C. albicans in vitro*.

Following the leucocyte transfusions, neither the magnitude of the response nor the antigen dose producing maximal stimulation were changed.

TABLE 3. Incorporation of tritiated thymidine by antigen and mitogen stimulated lymphocyte cultures from the patient, his father and healthy skin test-positive subjects

Antigen	Mean disintegrations per min				
	Patient	Father	Skin test positive normals		
			1	2	3
C. albicans sonicate					
0 (control)	1120	840	2040	4220	4000
50 μg/ml	780	865	1355	3570	1800
5 μg/ml	6330	15255	17640	27960	53700
0·5 μg/ml	5700	3240	4040	7620	7405
0·1 μg/ml	1030	239	1740	2700	1710
0·05 μg/ml	825	—	1200	—	—
Mumps					
0·1 ml	9490	—	10260	—	—
PHA-M					
0·1 ml	310770	507000	160500	99320	246000

Macrophage migration inhibition factor. Prior to the leucocyte transfusions, concentrated supernatants from the patient's antigen-stimulated lymphocytes did not inhibit migration of macrophages from capillary tubes (Table 4). In contrast, supernatant fluids from a Candida skin test positive subject, prepared under identical conditions, reduced the area of migration by 48·5%. Media containing the Candida extract in a concentration equal to the culture fluids did not impair migration of the macrophages.

TABLE 4. Macrophage migration-inhibition factor activity*

	Days following transfusion		
	Prior to transfusion	220	315
	% inhibition	% inhibition	% inhibition
Patient			
Supernatants from:			
unstimulated cultures	0	0	0
MEM plus Candida extract	0	0·7	−14·6
Candida stimulated cultures	3·0	20·7	9·3
Skin-Test Positive Control			
Supernantants from:			
unstimulated cultures	0	0	0
MEM plus Candida extract	0	0	−4·6
Candida stimulated cultures	48·5	20·5	28·9

* Each determination represents the mean of three chambers, each containing two capillary tubes.

181

An attempt to detect MIF activity in supernatants shortly after the leucocyte transfusion was a technical failure. When the study was repeated at 220 days, supernatants from Candida stimulated cells from the patient and control subject were equally effective in inhibiting migration from the capillary tubes. At 315 days, when the patient was in clinical relapse, and the delayed cutaneous reactions had reverted to negative, insignificant (9·3%) inhibition of migration was observed.

Immunoglobulins and serological findings. In contrast to abnormal cellular immunity, humoral responses of the patient were intact. The serum concentrations of the three major immunoglobulins were greater than normal (Table 5). Although IgE was not quantitatively

TABLE 5. Humoral immune responses and 'auto-antibodies' in the patient's serum

Serum Immunoglobulins	Normal range
IgG–25·6 mg/ml	5·0–12·0 γ/ml
IgA–7·2 mg/ml	1·5– 4·0 γ/ml
IgM–3·6 mg/ml	0·8– 3·0 γ/ml
IgE–present by skin test	
Candida Antibodies	
Serum agglutinins > 1:4096	
Salivary agglutinins 1:16	
Serum precipitins–positive	
Anti-A isoagglutinin 1:16	
'Auto-antibodies'	
anti-thyroglobulin 1:128	
anti-thyroid C-F 1:4	
anti-adrenal negative	
anti-gastric parietal	
cell negative	
rheumatoid factor (Latex) negative	
anti-nuclear factor negative	
cryoglobulin negative	

assayed, the wheal and flare reactions to Candida and SK-SD indicated the presence and function of this substance. Serum and saliva contained high titres of agglutinating antibodies against *C. albicans* (Table 5), and the serum contained precipitins against both mannans and cytoplasmic components of the yeast. Antibody activities against thyroglobulin and thyroid cells were found in the serum, but no other serological abnormalities were present.

Phagocytosis and inflammatory response. There were no abnormalities in the ability of the patient's peripheral leucocytes to ingest and kill staphylococci or *C. albicans*. Furthermore, the metabolic responses following phagocytosis as measured by increased activity of the pentose pathway and oxidation of formate, were normal. The patient's serum was found to opsonize *C. albicans* normally and histochemical stain for leucocyte peroxidase was positive.

Evolution of the inflammatory response as measured by the skin window technique of Rebuck & Crowley (1955) was normal.

TABLE 6. Leucocyte typing

	RBC Group	HL-A1	-A2	-A3	-A9	Lc17	-A5	-A7	-A8	HL-A12	TE 60 (Fiske)	Lc20
Patient	B	+	[+]	0	0	[0]	0	+	0	0	[0]	+
Father	B	+	[0]	0	0	[+]	0	+	0	0	[+]	+
Mother	A	0	+	0	0	0	0	0	0	0	0	0
Brother	0	0	0	0	0	+	0	0	0	0	+	0
Sister	0	0	0	0	0	+	0	0	0	0	+	0

* Mismatches involved in the leucocyte exchange are in square brackets.

Leucocyte and erythrocyte typing. The leucocyte antigens identified by the microdroplet cytotoxicity test are summarized on Table 6. None of the relatives were phenotypically identical with the patient. Furthermore, the mother and both siblings had different major erythrocyte antigens. The father, however, shared nineteen erythrocyte antigens with the patient, and possessed 's' which the patient lacked. Both leucocyte and erythrocyte cross-matches between the patient and his father were compatible.

Mixed leucocyte cultures also demonstrated the lack of HL-A identity in the family (Table 7). The magnitude of these responses was not altered when the cultures were incubated in autologous or homologous plasma. In the lower half of Table 7, the results of the reciprocal mixed leucocyte cultures are summarized and again brisk responses were found.

TABLE 7. Results of mixed leucocyte cultures

Responding cells	Stimulating cells			
	Self	Father	Mother	Sister
Patient	2170†	16900	10300	31850
Ratio*	1	7·8	4·7	14·7

Reciprocal Stimulation

Stimulating cells	Responding cells		
	Father	Mother	Sister
Self	1650	5180	2510
Patient	54950	83340	227650
Ratio*	33·3	16·1	90·7

* Mean dpm of response to allogenic cells divided by mean dpm of response to mitomycin treated autologous cells.
† Mean dpm from quadruplicate cultures.

Clinical responses following leucocyte transfusions. The evening following the third transfusion the patient became febrile and remained so for 48 hr. There were no other adverse effects.

During the ensuing months striking improvement was noted in the cutaneous lesions. This was especially apparent in areas that were not severely involved such as the scalp, neck (Fig. 1b), arms (Fig. 2b) and legs (Fig. 3b). More extensively affected areas such as the dorsum of the hands (Fig. 4b) also improved but to a lesser degree. There were no changes in the nails.

In the spring of 1970, approximately 8 months after the leucocyte transfusions, he noted recurrence of lesions in healed areas and exacerbation of areas with persistent infection. When he was studied in June, 1970, 10 months following the transfusions, the extent of the cutaneous lesions was similar to that of the previous year.

DISCUSSION

Despite its widespread natural occurrence and frequent presence in the human gastro-intestinal tract (Cohen *et al.*, 1970), severe infections due to *C. albicans* are uncommon. When systemic infections occur they are often in patients whose immune responses are impaired by malignancies (Hutter & Collins, 1962), immunosuppressive drugs (Rifkind *et al.*, 1967), or congenital defects of the thymus-dependent immune system such as the Di George syndrome, Nezeloff syndrome or lymphopenic agammaglobulinemia (Hermans *et al.*, 1969).

The mucocutaneous form of chronic moniliasis is unique in that it is limited to the mucous membranes, skin and nails, and essentially never involves parenchymal tissues. Reports containing several cases of this disorder illustrate the marked heterogeneity of the patient population in terms of age of onset, associated disorders such as polyendocrino-pathy, steatorrhea, and dental dysplasia, and immunological responses, especially delayed cutaneous hypersensitivity (Sjoberg, 1966; Chilgren *et al.*, 1967; Louria *et al.*, 1967; Blizzard & Cibbs, 1968; Hermans *et al.*, 1969; Kirkpatrick *et al.*, 1970). In view of the clinical variants of mucocutaneous moniliasis, it is not surprising that extensive studies have failed to define a defect in host-defence mechanisms that characterized all patients.

Abnormalities in phagocytic or metabolic properties of the patient's leucocytes similar to those reported by Lehrer & Cline (1969) were excluded by the normal ingestion and killing of *C. albicans*, and the normal increase in oxidation of glucose and formate following phagocytosis.

Attempts to alter the course of systemic Candida infections in animals with active or passive immunization have produced variable results (Dobias, 1964). Patients with muco-cutaneous moniliasis usually have normal or elevated titres of Candida antibodies in the serum and parotid fluid (Louria *et al.*, 1967; Kirkpatrick *et al.*, 1970) suggesting that humoral immune mechanisms are ineffective in resistance to this infection. A possible exception was described by Chilgren, and co-workers (1967), who reported two patients with mucocutaneous moniliasis and deficient Candida agglutinating antibodies in their parotid fluid IgA. These subjects also had negative cutaneous tests to Candida extracts, therefore their immunologic abnormality may involve the cellular immune system as well.

It is well known that addition of antigens to suspension cultures of sensitized peripheral blood lymphocytes induces biochemical and morphologic changes in a minor population of

184

the cells, and these *in vitro* responses correlate closely with delayed cutaneous hypersensitivity (Mills, 1966). When non-specific mitogens such as phytohemagglutinin or pokeweed mitogen are employed, the majority of the cells transform to 'blast-like' cells and undergo increased synthesis of DNA, RNA and protein (Ling, 1968). The cells that participate in these responses appear to be the 'thymus-dependent' small lymphocytes. Mitogen and antigen-induced lymphocyte transformation do not occur in cells from chicks that were thymectomized shortly after hatching (Greaves, Roitt & Rose, 1968), or with cells from infants born with a dysplastic or absent thymus (Lischner, Punnett & Di George, 1967).

Recently it has been shown that sensitized lymphocytes also respond to antigenic stimulation by releasing substances which inhibit migration of macrophages from capillary tubes (MIF) (David, 1968), are chemotactic for monocytes (Ward *et al.*, 1969), are cytotoxic (Granger & Williams, 1968) and recruit non-sensitized lymphocytes into DNA synthesis (Maini *et al.*, 1969; Kirkpatrick *et al.*, 1970). Injection of culture fluids containing MIF activity into the skin of normal animals produces histologic changes of delayed hypersensitivity (Bennett & Bloom, 1968) and it is generally believed that these 'mediators' are essential to the expression of cellular hypersensitivity.

Several reports of patients with chronic mucocutaneous moniliasis have noted negative delayed skin tests to *C. albicans* (Chilgren *et al.*, 1967; Louria *et al.*, 1967; Buckley *et al.*, 1968; Marmor & Barnett, 1968; Kirkpatrick *et al.*, 1970; Valdimarsson *et al.*, 1970). *In vitro* lymphocyte transformation studies have revealed that some patients with negative skin tests fail to respond to antigenic stimulation with an increase in thymidine incorporation (Chilgren *et al.*, 1967; Kirkpatrick *et al.*, 1970), while in others this response was normal (Chilgren *et al.*, 1967; Valdimarsson *et al.*, 1970). Chilgren *et al.* (1969) proposed that the latter group had a defect in production of mediators such as MIF. This hypothesis has been confirmed by Rocklin *et al.* (1970), Valdimarsson and co-workers (1970) and in the patient described in this report. Presumably these patients have antigen-sensitive peripheral blood lymphocytes that respond to *C. albicans* by replication, but are defective in the differentiative steps necessary for production or release of mediator substances.

The studies described here were directed toward defining the role of mediators in expression of delayed hypersensitivity, and evaluating the effect of an intact cellular immune system on the clinical course of chronic mucocutaneous moniliasis. It is clear that transfusions of large numbers of immunologically competent lymphoid cells were accompanied by conversion of the cutaneous response to *C. albicans* from negative to positive. During the months that the patient had reactive delayed cutaneous reactivity, supernatants from antigen-stimulated lymphocytes contained MIF activity. It is particularly significant that restoration of the immune response was accompanied by clinical improvement. While the patient had normal delayed hypersensitivity and mediator production, there was marked clearing of the cutaneous lesions. Furthermore, when an exacerbation of moniliasis occurred eight months after the cell transfusions, the skin tests had reverted to negative and no MIF was found in supernatants.

Studies of antibody synthesis (Claman & Chaperon, 1969) and graft-versus-host disease (Cantor & Asofsky, 1970) in rodents have demonstrated the synergistic relationships of cells from two different sources. Although both cells are probably bone marrow-derived, one type receives a differentiative influence from the thymus and becomes an antigen-sensitive cell. In mice, the other bone marrow-derived cell is independent of the thymus and becomes the precursor of the antibody synthesizing cell. Little is known about the nature of the interactions between these cells. Indeed, a mathematical analysis of the immune response to sheep erythrocytes in the mouse spleen has provided evidence for interactions involving three cell types (Mosier & Coppleson, 1968).

Studies of patients with chronic mucocutaneous moniliasis may provide evidence for multiple cell interactions in the expression of delayed hypersensitivity. For example, it is possible that a single antigen-sensitive peripheral lymphocyte responds to antigen by both mediator production and replication. Alternatively, the initial sensitizing experience may cause more primitive cells to differentiate into two lines, one that produces mediators in a manner analogous to antibody synthesis by plasma cells, and a second that responds by replication and serves to expand the pool of memory cells.

The findings in our patient could be explained by a defect in differentiation which did not affect cells with the capacity to replicate, but prohibited formation or function of the mediator producing cells. The transfusions of immuno-competent cells could have re-constituted this deficient or defective population and restored normal responsiveness. While it was not possible to document the duration of survival of the transfused allogenic cells, in man persistence of passively transferred delayed cutaneous hypersensitivity does not require the presence of viable donor cells. Lawrence (1969) has shown that 'transfer factor', released from sensitized lymphocytes by exposure to antigen or by lysis, is capable of transferring delayed cutaneous hypersensitivity specifically. Although not permanent, the transferred responses persist for months or years. The biological basis of its action is unknown. It is therefore possible that the cells transfused into our patient were rapidly destroyed and that the normal immune responses were mediated through transfer factor. Support for this possibility derives from the report of Rocklin *et al.* (1970), who found that MIF was produced by an anergic patient with moniliasis after treatment with transfer factor.

These studies support the earlier observations by Buckley *et al.* (1968) that reconstitution of the immune response may be useful in treating certain patients with chronic muco-cutaneous moniliasis. It is important to recognize that this disorder may occur in several settings and not all cases have presently definable abnormalities of the immune system. Under ideal circumstances, correction of the defect in appropriate patients would utilize matched lymphocytes or bone marrow in order to minimize the possibility of graft-versus-host reactions, or rejection of the graft. Alternative modes of therapy such as transfer factor also deserve consideration because they may correct the immune defect without the risk of sensitizing the patient to histocompatibility antigens, or producing adverse immune responses.

ACKNOWLEDGMENT

The authors are indebted to Dr Charles Pak for permission to study this patient and to Dr Herbert Hasenclever for providing mannans from *C. albicans*.

REFERENCES

BACH, F.H. & VOYNOW, N.K. (1966) One-way stimulation in mixed leukocyte cultures. *Science*, **153**, 545.

BENNETT, B. & BLOOM, B.R. (1968) Reactions *in vivo* and *in vitro* produced by a soluble substance associated with delayed-type hypersensitivity. *Proc. nat. Acad. Sci. (Wash.)* **59**, 756.

BLIZZARD, R.M. & GIBBS, J. H. (1968) Candidiasis: Studies pertaining to its association with endocrino-pathies and pernicious anemia. *Pediatrics*, **42**, 231.

BUCKLEY, R.H., LUCAS, Z.J., HATTLER, B.G. JR, ZMIJEWSKI, C.M. & AMOS, D.B. (1968) Defective cellular immunity associated with chronic mucocutaneous moniliasis and recurrent staphylococcal botryomycosis: Immunological reconstitution by allogenic bone marrow. *Clin. exp. Med.* **131**, 235.

BUCKNER, D., GRAW, R.G., EISEL, R.J., HENDERSON, E.S. & PERRY, S. (1969) Leukapheresis by continuous flow centrifugation (CFC) in patients with chronic myelogenous leukemia (CML). *Blood*, **33**, 353.

CANTOR, H. & ASOFSKY, R. (1970) Synergy among lymphoid cells mediating the graft versus-host-response. II. Synergy in graft-verusus-host reactions produced by Balb/c lymphoid cells of differing anatomic origin. *J. exp. Med.* **131**, 235.

CHILGREN, R.A., QUIE, P.G., MEUWISSEN, H.J. & HONG, R. (1967) Chronic mucocutaneous candidiasis, deficiency of delayed hypersensitivity and selective local antibody defect. *Lancet*, **ii**, 688.

CHILGREN, R.A., MEUWISSEN, H.J., QUIE, P.G., GOOD, R.A. & HONG, R. (1969) The cellular immune defect in chronic mucocutaneous moniliasis. *Lancet*, **i**, 1286.

CLAMAN, H.N. & CHAPERON, E.A. (1969) Immunologic complementation between thymus and marrow cells—a model for the two-cell theory of immunocompetence. *Transplant. Rev.* **1**, 92.

CLEVELAND, W.W., FOGEL, B.J., BROWN, W.T. & KAY, H.E.M. (1968) Foetal thymic transplant in a case of Di George's syndrome. *Lancet*, **ii**, 1211.

COHEN, R., ROTH, F.J., DELGADO, E., AHERN, D.G. & KALSER, M.H. (1969) Fungal flora of the normal human small and large intestine. *New Engl. J. Med.* **280**, 638.

DAVID, J.R. (1968) Macrophage migration. *Fed. Proc.* **27**, 6.

DOBIAS, B. (1964) Specific and nonspecific immunity to Candida infections: Experimental studies of role of Candida cell constituents and review of literature. *Acta. med. scand.* **176**, suppl. 42, 1.

GRANGER, G.A. & WILLIAMS, T.W. (1968) Lymphocyte cytotoxicity *in vitro*: Activation and release of a cytotoxic factor. *Nature (Lond.)*, **218**, 1253.

GREAVES, M.F., ROITT, I.M. & ROSE, M.E. (1968) Effect of bursectomy and thymectomy on the responses of chicken peripheral blood lymphocytes to phytohemagglutinin. *Nature (Lond.)*, **220**, 293.

HERMANS, P.F., ULRICH, J.A. & MARKOWITZ, H. (1969) Chronic mucocutaneous candidiasis as a surface expression of deep seated abnormalities. *Amer. J. Med.* **47**, 503.

HUTTER, R.V.P. & COLLINS, H.S. (1962) The occurrence of opportunistic fungal infections in a cancer hospital. *Lab. Invest.* **11**, 1035.

KIRKPATRICK, C.H., CHANDLER, J.W., JR & SCHIMKE, R.N. (1970) Chronic mucocutaneous moniliasis with impaired delayed hypersensitivity. *Clin. exp. Immunol.* **6**, 375.

KIRKPATRICK, C.H., STITES, D.P., SMITH, T.K. & JOHNSON, R.A. (1970) A factor which enhances DNA synthesis in cultures of stimulated lymphocytes, *Proceedings of the Fourth Leukocyte Culture Conference* (Ed. by O. R. McIntyre) p. 219. Appleton-Century-Crofts, New York.

LAWRENCE, H.S. (1969) Transfer factor. *Adv. Immunol.* Vol. 11 (Ed. by F. J. Dixon and H. G. Kunkel), p. 195. Academic Press, New York.

LEHRER, R.I. & CLINE, M.J. (1969) Leukocyte myeloperoxidase deficiency and disseminated candidiasis: the role of myeloperoxidase in resistance to Candida infection. *J. clin. Invest.* **48**, 1478.

LING, N.R. (1968) *Lymphocyte Stimulation*, p. 147. North Holland Publishing Co., Amsterdam.

LISCHNER, H.W., PUNNETT, H.H. & DI GEORGE, A.M. (1967) Lymphocytes in congenital absence of the thymus. *Nature (Lond.)*, **214**, 580.

LOURIA, D.B., SHANNON, D., JOHNSON, G., CAROLINE, L., OKAS, A. & TASCHDJIAN, C. (1967) The susceptibility to moniliasis in children with endocrine hypofunction. *Trans. Assoc. Amer. Physicians*, **80**, 236.

MAINI, R.N., BRYCESON, A.D.M., WOLSTENCROFT, R.A. & DUMONDE, D.C. (1969) Lymphocyte mitogenic factor in man. *Nature (Lond.)*, **224**, 43.

MANCINI, G., CARBONARA, A.O. & HEREMANS, J.F. (1965) Immuno-chemical quantitation of antigens by single radial immunodiffusion. *Immunochemistry* **2**, 235.

MARMOR, M.F. & BARNETT, E.V. (1968) Cutaneous anergy without systemic disease. *Amer. J. Med.* **44**, 979.

MICKENBERG, I.D., ROOT, R.K. & WOLFF, S.M. (1970) Leukocyte function in hypogammaglobulinemia. *J. clin. Invest.* **49**, 1528.

MILLS, J.A. (1966) The immunologic significance of antigen induced lymphocyte transformation *in vitro*. *J. Immunol.* **97**, 239.

MITTAL, K.K., MICKEY, M.R., SINGAL, D.P. & TERASAKI, P.I. (1968) Serotyping for transplantation. XVIII. Refinement of microdroplet lymphocyte cytotoxicity test. *Transplantation*, **6**, 913.

187

Mosier, D.E. & Coppleson, L.W. (1968) A three-cell interaction required for the induction of the primary immune response *in vitro*. *Proc. nat. Acad. Sci.* (*Wash.*), **61**, 542.

Newberry, M.W., Chandler, J.W. Jr, Chin, T.D.Y. & Kirkpatrick, C.H. (1968) Immunology of the myoses. I. Depressed lymphocyte transformation in chronic histoplasmosis. *J. Immunol.* **100**, 436.

Ouchterlony, O. (1962) Diffusion-in-gel methods for immunologic analysis. Prog. Allergy, Vol. 6 (Ed. by P. Kallos and B. H. Waksman), p. 30. S. Karger, New York.

Rebuck, J.W. & Crowley, J.H. (1955) A method of studying leukocytic functions *in vivo*. *Ann. N.Y. Acad. Sci.* **59**, 757.

Rifkind, D., Marchioro, T.L., Schneck, S.A. & Hill, R.B., Jr (1967) Systemic fungal infections complicating renal transplantation and immunosuppressive therapy. *Amer. J. Med.* **43**, 28.

Rocklin, R.E., Meyers, O.L. & David, J.R. (1970) An *in vitro* assay for cellular hypersensitivity in man. *J. Immunol.* **104**, 95.

Rocklin, R.E., Chilgren, R.A., Hong, R. & David, J.R. (1970) Transfer of cellular hypersensitivity in chronic mucocutaneous candidiasis monitored *in vivo* and *in vitro*. *Cell. Immunol.* **1**, 290.

Sjoberg, K.H. (1966) Moniliasis—an internal disease? *Acta med. scand.* **179**, 157.

Thor, D.E., Jureziz, R.E., Veach, S.R., Miller, E. & Dray, S. (1968) Cell migration inhibition factor released by antigen from human peripheral lymphocytes. *Nature* (*Lond.*), **219**, 755.

Valdimarsson, H., Holt, L., Riches, H.R.C. & Hobbs, J.R. (1970) Lymphocyte abnormality in chronic mucocutaneous candidiasis. *Lancet*, i, 1259.

Ward, P.A., Remold, H.G. & David, J.R. (1969) Leukotactic factor produced by sensitized lymphocytes. *Science*, **163**, 1079.

THYMUS TRANSPLANTATION

Permanent Reconstitution of Cellular Immunity in a Patient with Sex-Linked Combined Immunodeficiency

ARTHUR J. AMMANN, M.D., DIANE W. WARA, M.D., SYDNEY SALMON, M.D., AND HERBERT PERKINS, M.D.

Abstract Successful reconstitution of cell-mediated immunity was achieved in a four-week-old infant with sex-linked severe combined immunodeficiency by intraperitoneal transplantation of a 14-week gestational-age fetal thymus. Ten days after transplantation, a new HL-A antigen was detected in the infant that was present in the mother of the thymus donor. Two months after transplantation, the patient's total lymphocyte count was normal. At four months, three of the pre-transplant HL-A antigens were not detectable, and three antigens of the mother of the thymus donor were present. Nine months after transplantation, the patient's in vitro phytohemagglutinin response and pokeweed mitogen response were normal. Immunologic reconstitution in this patient was probably achieved by lymphocyte repopulation, as evidenced by the length of time required for normal cell-mediated immune responses to develop, and by the development of lymphocyte HL-A chimerism.

TRANSPLANTATION of fetal thymus resulting in permanent reconstitution of cellular immunity has been accomplished only in the DiGeorge syndrome.[1,2] Temporary reconstitution has been achieved in various immunodeficiency diseases associated with thymic hypoplasia.[3,4]

Recently, we transplanted a fetal thymus to a four-week-old infant with severe combined immunodeficiency. A mild graft-versus-host reaction was observed. Subsequently, gradual improvement in cell-mediated immunity occurred. Currently, the patient is 18 months of age and has normal cell-mediated immunity but absent antibody-mediated immunity.

Supported by a grant (5MO1-RR00079-10) from the Division of Research Resources, National Institutes of Health, by grants (NIAID71-2203 and 72-2500) from the National Institute of Allergy and Infectious Diseases, by the John Hartford Foundation and by grants (CA 14087 and Ca 11067) from the National Institutes of Health.

189

CASE PRESENTATION

Family History

The maternal great-grandmother had 6 children: 2 sons died in infancy from unknown causes, 1 son was chronically ill and 3 daughters were normal. A maternal aunt had 4 children: 3 sons died within the 1st 4 months of life from infection, and a 4th received gamma globulin for a brief time but is now normal (a diagnosis of hypogammaglobulinemia was never established). Another maternal aunt had 5 children: 4 daughters were normal, and 1 son died at 5 months of age with progressive vaccinia and graft-versus-host reaction. At autopsy he had a thymus that weighed 1.5 g and lacked Hassall's corpuscles and corticomedullary differentiation. There was marked depletion of lymphoid tissue. The case is reported in detail in two separate publications.[5,6]

Patient History

The patient was the 1st-born child. Because of a family history suggestive of sex-linked severe combined immunodeficiency, a chest x-ray study and total lymphocyte count were obtained immediately after birth. No thymic shadow was seen, and lymphopenia was present (Table 1). Physical examination gave normal results. He was kept in a bassinet that was placed in a laminar flow hood (Pure Air Corporation); he was maintained in this atmosphere until evaluation and therapy were completed.

Initial studies included immunization with antibody to pneumococcal polysaccharide (Types I, III, IV, VII, VIII and XII), quantitative immunoglobulins and response of isolated peripheral lymphocytes in vitro to phytohemagglutinin and mixed leukocyte culture (Table 1). Evaluation and family history led to a diagnosis of sex-linked severe combined immunodeficiency.

The infant continued to do well except for the onset of tinea corporis at 2 weeks of age.

Because there were no siblings and, therefore, no potential donors of histocompatible bone marrow, transfer-factor therapy was attempted. No evidence of immunologic reconstitution was observed. The total volume of blood required for repeated blood studies resulted in moderate anemia. After radiation with 3,000 R, 40 ml of blood was administered. At 4 weeks of age, a fetal thymus was transplanted. One week later, the tinea lesion, which had been resistant to local antifungal therapy and was spreading rapidly before the thymus transplant, cleared competely. A maculopapular rash — similar to that seen in early graft-versus-host reactions — was now present over the entire body. Repeat immunologic studies gave no evidence of reconstitution. At 7 weeks of age, rapid, grunting respirations with some worsening of the skin rash developed. Hair loss, jaundice, diarrhea and hepatosplenomegaly were not observed. Liver enzymes remained normal. However, lymphopenia became more severe (count of 1420) and was associated with thrombocytopenia. At 8 weeks of age, diffuse superficial desquamation in the areas of the rash was observed. A skin biopsy of the rash showed mononuclear infiltration surrounding the blood vessels of the dermis. The rash gradually cleared, and the patient was discharged at 9 weeks of age. He was given gamma-globulin injections and followed at monthly intervals until the present. No attempt was made to isolate the infant, and he remained entirely well until the age of 14 months, when vomiting, diarrhea and dehydration developed. Salmonella Group C was cultured from the stool. Blood and spinal-fluid cultures were sterile.

190

Table 1. Data on Antibody and Cell-Mediated Immunity.*

Age	Therapy	Quantitative Immunoglobulins (Mg/100 Ml)			Antibody (Fold Increase)		Total Lymphocyte Count (Mm³)	Phytohemagglutinin Response in Vitro		Mixed Lymphocyte Culture in Vitro†	
		IgG	IgM	IgA	PPS	KLH		stimulated cpm/nonstimulated cpm	index	response	index
Birth		1400	0	0	0	ND					
3 wk					0	ND					
3½ wk							2418	439/1737	0.3	61/77	0.8
4 wk	Transfer factor				0	ND					
4½ wk	Thymus transplant						2247	174/1483	0.1		
1 wk after transplant							2480	584/123	5		
2 mo after transplant		320	16	0	0	0	3600	2686/2662	1		
4 mo after transplant		180	13	0	0	0	5890	2041/709	3		
9 mo after transplant		210	10	0	0	0	3038	18,456/234	79	2145/15.6	138

*ND represents not done, PPS pneumococcal polysaccharide, & KLH keyhole-limpet hemocyanin.

†Mixed lymphocyte culture response in vitro: patient responding against mother/patient mitomycin treated against mother mitomycin treated.

He was treated with intravenous ampicillin and responded well. Therapy was discontinued. At the age of 18 months he remained well; however, stool cultures continued to contain salmonella.

Laboratory studies indicate gradual reconstitution of cell-mediated immunity (Table 1) associated with a repopulation of the patient by lymphocytes from the thymus donor (Table 2).

MATERIALS AND METHODS

Serum immunoglobulins were quantitated by single radial diffusion with use of a modification of the Mancini technic and the World Health Organization reference serums for standardization.

The patient was immunized with 50 μg of hexavalent pneumococcal polysaccharide (Types I, III, IV, VII, VIII and XII) obtained from the National Institute of Allergy and Infectious Diseases (produced by Eli Lilly and Company) and with 50 μg of keyhole-limpet hemocyanin (Pacific Bio-Marine Supply Company). Antibody titers were measured by indirect hemagglutination and were compared before and 2 weeks after immunization.[7]

In vitro reactivity of lymphocytes to phytohemagglutinin (Burroughs Wellcome) was measured by addition of 0.5 μg of phytohemagglutinin per milliliter of culture medium or 1 μg of phytohemagglutinin per milliliter of culture medium containing 2×10^6 isolated lymphocytes per milliliter. All cultures were run in triplicate and were run simultaneously with nonstimulated control cultures. Cultures were incubated for 96 hours: ^{14}C-thymidine; 0.1 mCi, was added to the cells and incubated for an additional 16 hours. DNA was then precipitated, solubilized and counted in a scintillation counter. Normal control lymphocytes activated with phytohemagglutinin incorporated 50 to 400 times more ^{14}C-thymidine than the unstimulated cells. Identical methodology was used to evaluate reactivity of lymphocytes to keyhole-limpet hemocyanin, pokeweed mitogen and mixed leukocyte culture[8] except that 5-day incubation periods were used. Keyhole-limpet hemocyanin, 5 to 15 μg per milliliter of cell suspension, elicited 20 times more ^{14}C-thymidine incorporation in stimulated than in unstimulated cells.[9]

Table 2. HL-A Phenotypes.

SUBJECT	LA LOCUS		4 LOCUS		FACTORS INCOMPATIBLE WITH INHERITANCE
Father	HL-A2	—	HL-A5	H1-A12	
Mother	HL-A2	HL-A3	HL-A7	W18	
Mother's sister	HL-A3	HL-A10	HL-A5	HL-A7	
Mother of thymus donor	HL-A11	W19	HL-A5	W22	
Patient:					
Before transplant	HL-A2	HL-A3	HL-A7	HL-A12	
10 days after transplant	HL-A2	HL-A3	HL-A7	HL-A12	W19
20 days after transplant	HL-A2	HL-A3	HL-A7	HL-A12	W19
4 mo after transplant	Negative	Negative	HL-A7	Negative	W19, W22, HL-A11

The patient's lymphocytes (1×10^6 per milliliter), both mitomy-cin-C-treated and untreated, were incubated with normal treated and untreated lymphocytes (1×10^6 per milliliter) in culture. Un-treated control cells in mixed lymphocyte culture incorporated 50 times more ^{14}C-thymidine than treated control cells.

HL-A typing and screening for antibodies were performed by the fluorochromasia cytotoxicity technic of Bodmer.[10] The number of serum samples used to detect each HL-A factor of importance in this case was as follows: HL-A2, 6; HL-A3, 5; HL-A11, 7; W19, 10; HL-A7, 13; HL-A12, 9; and W22, 5. Each typing was repeated on a separate occasion for confirmation.

Transfer factor was prepared from 1 U of blood obtained from a donor who was skin-test positive to mumps, candida and streptoki-nase-streptodornase. It was prepared by the method of Lawrence and administered intramuscularly.[11]

The thymus transplant was performed with a thymus gland ob-tained from a 14-week fetus. The mother was clinically well and un-derwent therapeutic abortion by hysterotomy. The thymus was maintained in physiologic saline at ambient temperature for 2 hours before transplant. It was dissected out, minced and transplanted in-traperitoneally via a 16-gauge intracatheter.

RESULTS

Table 1 represents the accumulated data on anti-body and cell-mediated immunity in the patient be-fore and after transplantation. Values of IgG, which were normal at birth, fell steadily and were maintained at approximately 200 mg per 100 ml by monthly gamma-globulin injections. Some IgM was synthe-sized, but no IgA was detected. No antibody response to pneumococcal polysaccharide was detected before or after transfer factor or before or after thymus transplantation. No antibody to keyhole-limpet hemo-cyanin was detected after thymus transplantation.

Cell-mediated immunity, which was absent at birth and after administration of transfer factor, was first im-portant by in vitro lymphocyte response to phytohem-agglutinin four months after thymus transplantation. Cell-mediated immunity was normal nine months after transplantation when assayed by total lympho-cyte count (3038), lymphocyte response in vitro to phytohemagglutinin (stimulation index of 79) and pokeweed mitogen (stimulation index of 29). Mixed lymphocyte culture was assayed 11 months after transplantation and was normal. However, delayed hypersensitivity as detected by a battery of skin tests re-mained absent. Thymus shadow continued to be ab-sent on chest x-ray study.

Table 2 presents evidence based on HL-A pheno-types of the patient. Four HL-A antigens consistent with inheritance from his parents were unequivocally present until four months after transplantation. In addition, 10 days after transplantation, a new HL-A antigen (W19) was first detected that was present in the phenotype of the mother of the thymus donor. Four months after transplantation, the inherited factors HL-A2, HL-A3 and HL-A12 were no longer detectable on his peripheral blood lymphocytes, but HL-A11, W19 and W22 were unequivocally present. Lymphocytes from the mother of the thymus donor (typed by Dr. Paul Terasaki) revealed that she had HL-A11, W19 and W22 in common with the patient's sample four months after transplantation. Dr. Terasaki also typed the patient's cells nine months after transplantation. He confirmed the presence of HL-A11 and W22 but detected no other antigens. These results probably indicate that the cells being typed from the blood of the patient were cells of the thymus donor, who had inherited either the HL-A11, W22, or the W19, W22, haplotype from his mother. The donor's father was not available for typing.

Further evidence of change in HL-A typing was obtained from antibody studies. Table 3 shows that initially the mother possessed an antibody that reacted

Table 3. Cytotoxic Antibodies for Lymphocytes.

PERIOD OF STUDY	LYMPHOCYTES				
	PANEL	FATHER'S	MOTHER'S	PATIENT'S 10 DAYS AFTER TRANSPLANT	PATIENT'S 4 MO AFTER TRANSPLANT
Mother's serum:					
10 days after transplant	+7/10	+		+	Negative
5 wk after transplant				+	Negative
4 mo after transplant	+8/10				
5 mo after transplant	+4/10		Negative	+	Negative
Patient's serum:					
3 wk before transplant	+0/9	+	Negative	Negative	
2 wk before transplant	+1/9	+	Negative	Negative	
Day of transplant	+7/10	±	±	Negative	
10 days after transplant	+7/20	±	+	Negative	
3 wk after transplant	+6/10	+	+	Negative	
4 mo after transplant	+6/10	Negative	Negative		

both with the lymphocytes of the father and with the lymphocytes of the patient 10 days after transplantation. The mother's initial serum, tested simultaneously, did not react with the infant's cells obtained four months after transplantation; at this time his cells had lost three of their original HL-A factors (Table 2). In addition, he initially had a weak antibody reacting with his father's cells that had disappeared by four months after transplantation (Table 3). This development probably represents passive transfer of antibody from the mother.

Discussion

A diagnosis of sex-linked severe combined immunodeficiency disease was established by a suggestive family history with a previous case report in a male cousin who had characteristic features of deficient antibody and cell-mediated immunity, graft-versus-host reaction and progressive vaccinia,[5,6] and also by deficient antibody-mediated and cell-mediated immunity on laboratory testing of the patient. Because there were no siblings who could serve as possible HL-A-compatible bone-marrow donors, treatment with transfer factor and thymus transplantation was planned. No evidence of immunologic reconstitution was found after transfer-factor administration.

Subsequent transplantation of a 14-week-old fetal thymus did not result in immediate evidence of reconstitution. The earliest evidence of an effect of the thymus transplant occurred within seven days, with a clearing of a tinea lesion that had been resistant to all forms of topical therapy. The clearing occurred shortly before the appearance of a diffuse maculopapular rash typical of a graft-versus-host reaction; although all the manifestations of such a reaction were not observed, increased lymphopenia, thrombocytopenia, a skin biopsy showing mononuclear-cell infiltration of the dermis and subsequent desquamation in areas of the rash were consistent with a diagnosis of mild graft-versus-host reaction. In addition, HL-A chimerism was demonstrated. This finding contradicts previous observations concerning the ability of fetal thymus transplants to produce a graft-versus-host reaction.[12] It may be that the host is a more important determinant in such reactions than the age of the fetal thymus. We have used 20-week-old fetal thymus to transplant into children with thymic hypoplasia syndromes, without evidence of subsequent graft-versus-host reactions. In thymic hypoplasia syndromes, it is likely that reconstitution is the consequence of a thymic humoral factor that restores the patient's own immunity and results in rejection of the transplant.

In contrast with the rapid restoration of cell-mediated immunity observed in patients with the DiGeorge syndrome and thymic hypoplasia,[1-4] normal cell-mediated immunity did not develop in our patient until nine months after thymus transplant. The rapid reconstitution of cell-mediated immunity (three to five days after thymus transplantation) and the lack of chimerism demonstrated in patients with the DiGeorge syndrome and thymic hypoplasia suggests reconstitution by a humoral factor whereas the slow reconstitution associated with HL-A chimerism in the present case suggests reconstitution by cellular repopulation.

Before transplantation, all HL-A antigens could be accounted for on the basis of inheritance. Afterward, antigens were observed in addition to the patient's own. Four months after transplantation, three of the original HL-A antigens were no longer detectable and were replaced by three HL-A antigens represented in the phenotype of the mother of the thymus donor. (Testing for white-cell chimerism by sex chromosomes was not possible since the thymus donor was a male.) It is unlikely that the chimerism demonstrated represented the phenomenon of "spurious" antigens reported in some patients with combined immunodeficiency disease.[13,14] Extra antigens were not found before transplantation and those found subsequently could be accounted for on the basis of transplantation. Additional evidence for reconstitution by fetal thymus is obtained from an analysis of cytotoxic antibodies in the patient's mother (Table 3). Simultaneous testing of the mother's serum against the patient's cells obtained 10 days and four months after transplantation revealed the presence of antibodies cytotoxic for the infant cells obtained 10 days but absent cytotoxicity against infant cells obtained four months after transplantation. The change in cytotoxicity correlates with the most marked change in HL-A-antigen typing.

Definite evidence of reconstitution of cell-mediated immunity was not observed until four months after transplantation, when a total lymphocyte count of 5890 was achieved. This was associated with a positive although subnormal phytohemagglutinin response four months after transplantation. On re-evaluation nine months after transplantation, the patient's total lymphocyte count, phytohemagglutinin response and pokeweed-mitogen response were normal. Two months later the mixed lymphocyte response was normal. Only the response to antigen sensitization (keyhole-limpet hemocyanin) was absent (tested in vivo by delayed hypersensitivity and in vitro by lymphocyte stimulation).

There was no evidence for reconstitution of antibody-mediated immunity. On repeated testing, immunoglobulin quantitation revealed no IgA, IgM of 10 to 16 mg per 100 ml and a recent IgG of 210 mg per 100 ml during gamma-globulin therapy. Immunization with a thymic-independent antigen (pneumococcal polysaccharide) and a thymic-dependent antigen (keyhole-limpet hemocyanin) resulted in no detectable antibody response.

The restoration of all measured indexes of cell-mediated immunity except in vivo and in vitro cell-mediated immune response to keyhole-limpet hemocyanin suggests that an essential component, lacking in fetal thymus, may be necessary for complete reconstitution.

The lack of successful reconstitution in previous cases of combined immunodeficiency disease by means of thymus transplantation may be explained on the basis of concomitant systemic infection and death before establishment of immunity. Our patient was entirely well at the time of transplantation and remained well until the first evidence of cell-mediated immunity was detected. The technic of thymus transplantation may also be important. In this case the thymus was transplanted intraperitoneally within two hours after abortion. In contrast, in previous reports the thymus was usually transplanted intramuscularly by surgical means after long periods between abortion and transplantation.[15] In other cases, frozen thymus was used. These methods may have resulted in a definite decrease in cell viability.

References

1. August CS, Rosen FS, Filler RM, et al: Implantation of a foetal thymus: restoring immunological competence in a patient with thymic aplasia (DiGeorge's syndrome). Lancet 2:1210-1211, 1968
2. Cleveland WW, Fogel BJ, Brown WY, et al: Foetal thymic transplant in a case of DiGeorge's syndrome. Lancet 2:1211-1214, 1968
3. Levy R, Huang J, Bach ML, et al: Thymic transplantation in a case of chronic mucocutaneous candidiasis. Lancet 2:898-900, 1971
4. Hong R, Huang SW, Levy R, et al: Cartilage-hair hypoplasia: effect of thymus transplants. Clin Immunol Immunopathol 1:15-26, 1972
5. Fulginiti VA, Kempe CH, Hathaway WE, et al: Progressive vaccinia in immunologically deficient individuals, Immunologic Deficiency Diseases in Man (Birth Defects Original Article Series, Vol 4, No 1). Edited by D Bergsma. New York, The National Foundation, 1968, pp 129-146
6. Hathaway WE, Githens JH, Blackburn WR, et al: Aplastic anemia, his-

tiocytosis and erythrodermia in immunologically deficient children: probable human runt disease. N Engl J Med 273:953-965, 1965

7. Ammann AJ, Pelger RJ: Determination of antibody to pneumococcal polysaccharides with chromic chloride-treated human red blood cells and indirect hemagglutination. Appl Microbiol 24:679-683, 1972

8. Bach FH, Voynow NK: One-way stimulation in mixed leukocyte cultures. Science 153:545-547, 1966

9. Curtis JE, Hersh EM, Butler WT, et al: Antigen dose in the human immune response: dose-response relationships in the human immune response to Keyhole limpet hemocyanin. J Lab Clin Med 78:61-69, 1971

10. Bodmer W, Tripp M, Bodmer J: Application of a fluorochromatic cytotoxicity assay to human leukocyte typing, Histocompatibility Testing. 1967. Edited by ES Curtoni, PL Mattiuz, RM Tosi. Copenhagen, Ejnar Munksgaard, 1967, p 341

11. Lawrence HS, Al-Askari S: The preparation and purification of transfer factor, In Vitro Methods in Cell-Mediated Immunity. Edited by BR Bloom, PR Glade. New York, Academic Press, 1971, pp 531-546

12. Buckley RH: Reconstitution: grafting of bone marrow and thymus, Progress in Immunology: First International Congress of Immunology. Edited by B Amos. New York, Academic Press, 1971, pp 1061-1080

13. Sanderson AR, Gelfand EQ, Rosen FS: A change in HL-A phenotype associated with a specific blocking factor in the serum of an infant with severe combined immunodeficiency disease. Transplantation 13:142-145, 1972

14. Terasaki PI, Miyajima T, Sengar DPS, et al: Extraneous lymphocytic HL-A antigens in severe combined immunodeficiency disease. Transplantation 13:250-255, 1972

15. Githens JH, Fulginiti VA, Suvatte E, et al: Grafting of fetal thymus and hematopoietic tissue in infants with immune deficiency syndromes. Transplantation (in press)

198

Histopathology of *Mycobacterium bovis* (BCG)-Mediated Tumor Regression[1,2]

M. G. Hanna, Jr., M. J. Snodgrass, Berton Zbar, *and* Herbert J. Rapp.

SUMMARY—A comparative histopathologic study was performed on inbred guinea pigs at the site of a transplanted syngeneic hepatocarcinoma and in the draining lymph nodes, in the presence and absence of *Mycobacterium bovis* strain bacillus Calmette-Guérin (BCG). BCG was injected into the growing intradermal tumor 7 days after transplantation when the tumor had metastasized to the first regional lymph node. The histopathology was compared with that of saline-inoculated tumors and with that of animals in which tumors had been surgically removed 7 days after transplantation. In this system guinea pigs died 60–90 days after intradermal injection of 10^6 hepatocarcinoma cells without BCG treatment. The results demonstrate that intradermal tumors completely regress after treatment with BCG and that regional lymph node metastases are eliminated. The mechanism is a BCG-mediated granulomatous reaction at both the tumor site and the regional lymph node. As detected histologically and ultrastructurally, histiocytes appear to be the major effector cells in this reaction. In this syngeneic tumor system, conventional lymphoproliferative response of the regional node, in the absence of histiocytosis, is insufficient to inhibit tumor growth. Additionally, treatment of these transplanted syngeneic tumors in guinea pigs with a single sensitization by vaccinia virus, oxazolone, or turpentine was compared with BCG therapy. Cellular reactions in the regional lymph nodes, which were characteristic of the development of delayed-type hypersensitivity, were not detrimental to the tumor and did not alter metastatic growth. The turpentine-induced inflammatory reaction at the tumor site was also ineffective in suppressing tumor growth. Both turpentine and oxazolone treatments, however, enhanced tumor growth in the skin.

AN EXPERIMENTAL MODEL consisting of a transplantable syngeneic hepatocarcinoma in inbred guinea pigs has been developed to study the requirements of effective cancer immunotherapy (*1*). Studies with this model have demonstrated that

[1] Presented at Conference on Immunology of Carcinogenesis, held by the Oak Ridge National Laboratory at Gatlinburg, Tenn., May 8–11, 1972.

[2] Research supported jointly by the National Cancer Institute and by the U.S. Atomic Energy Commission under contract with the Union Carbide Corporation.

nonimmunized animals challenged with living tumor cells before treatment can be cured by active immunization only if the number of tumor cells in the challenge inoculum is relatively small and the interval between challenge and treatment is short enough so that a palpable tumor is not present at the time of treatment (2).

In another approach, inbred male guinea pigs (Sewall-Wright strain 2) with palpable intradermal tumors and metastases in the lymph node draining the tumor site can be permanently cured by the injection of living *Mycobacterium bovis* bacillus Calmette-Guérin (BCG) into the skin tumor (3). In this experimental model, untreated guinea pigs die 60–90 days after intradermal injection of 1×10^6 line-10 syngeneic hepatocarcinoma cells. Evidence has been presented indicating that nonlymphoid mononuclear cells are important in the process leading to tumor regression (4, 5). This report deals with a study of the histopathology of the site of the regressing tumor and the draining lymph node.

HISTOPATHOLOGY OF TUMOR REGRESSION AFTER BCG INJECTION

Of paramount importance in understanding the mechanism of BCG-mediated tumor and metastasis regression is the histopathology of the events of the tuberculin reaction in the tumor site and the draining lymph node. These results will be of more than just academic interest, since as described recently by Spector (6), the histology of the host response to tubercle bacilli is still the subject of debate. The cutaneous reaction to living BCG appears essentially to be a biphasic inflammatory response, consisting of an immediate (polymorphonuclear) reaction followed by a vigorous mononuclear response. The hematogenous origin of the mononuclear cell in the reaction site can be assumed, based on studies by Kosunen et al. (7) and Volkman and Gowans (8) in normal animals. These cells have been generally classified as macrophages of monocytic origin, derived from the bone marrow (9).

We evaluated the histopathology at the skin site

(upper right quadrant) of a transplanted syngeneic hepatocarcinoma and in the draining lymph node in the presence and absence of *Mycobacterium bovis* strain BCG (Phipps strain TMC 1029). Twenty-four $\times$ 10^6 living BCG were injected into the intradermal tumor 7 days after transplantation, a time suspected to be the earliest stage of metastasis to the draining lymph node. The histopathology was compared to that of saline-inoculated tumors and to that of animals in which tumors had been excised at day 7. Normal guinea pigs receiving a single intradermal BCG injection were also evaluated as controls (*10*).

It is important to qualify the terminology to be associated with these descriptions, because of the difficulty of interpreting the extensive literature on classic tuberculin granulomatous disease. The general term histiocyte is used to refer to a cell type distinguishable from active macrophages or phagocytic mononuclear cells and consistent with the characteristics of the epitheloid cells associated with granulomatous reactions (*11*). It is accepted that these may be different forms of the same cell type (*12*). Also, it is recognized that in the early host response, phagocytosis of a limited number of bacilli by macrophages initially activates this cell compartment, as described by Dannenberg (*13*). However, the general absence of active phagocytosis and representative numbers of cell inclusion bodies in the enlarged, activated compartment of responding cells tends to argue against phagocytosis as their sole primary function. We reject the terms "epithelioid" and "epithelial-like cell" because they are based on a superficial resemblance and are misleading with respect to the origin and function of the cell.

Tumor Site and Lymph Node Before Treatment

Histologic examination 4 days after tumor cell injection showed tumor cells to be confined to the skin. They were retained within the reticular layer of the dermis, with subcutaneous extension.

The chain of lymph nodes draining the tumor site were carefully selected and examined histo-

201

logically and ultrastructurally. The first ipsilateral node was the superficial distal axillary (SDA) lymph node. Anterior to this was the proximal axillary (PA) lymph node. Similar dissection was performed on the contralateral side. Both the SDA and PA lymph nodes, the first and second nodes draining this tumor site, were free of tumor cells and appeared normal at 4 days. These nodes possessed intact nodular cortical (thymus-independent) and paracortical (thymus-dependent) regions and occasional germinal centers in the nodules of the cortical zone. The marginal sinus surrounded the cortex, and we considered that the population of cells of the marginal sinus represented cells from the afferent lymph. A normal medulla consisted of both cords and sinuses (fig. 1).

By day 7 the tumor had grown mainly within the subcutaneous regions of the skin, and a slight mononuclear cell infiltration consisting of lymphocytes and occasional histiocytes surrounded the penetrating edge of the tumor mass. Tumor cells could be observed in the SDA lymph node at 7 days. The tumor cells, both intact and in mitosis, were confined to the subcapsular marginal sinus (fig. 2). Thus it was established that metastasis had occurred in the first draining node before treatment or excision of the tumor. No evidence of metastasis could be observed in any other lymph nodes of either the ipsilateral or contralateral side.

Comparison of Saline or BCG Intralesional Injection and Tumor Excision

One day after saline injection, mononuclear cells infiltrated the subcutaneous border of the tumor. This infiltration consisted mainly of lymphocytes and occasional histiocytes. At day 4 after saline injection (day 11 after tumor cell injection) the tumor mass had visibly increased in size without quantitative or qualitative change of mononuclear cell infiltration. At 25 days after saline injection there was a massive tumor growth (fig. 3) and a marked increase in the associated connective tissue component of the skin. Whether this is a characteristic of the tumor mass or a response of the local connective tissue to the invading tumor is undeci-

202

ded. Also, within the tumor mass there was a deep infiltration of lymphocytes and occasional histiocytes.

In contrast to the tumor site alterations after saline injection, 24 hours after BCG injection an acute inflammatory reaction was observed in the tumor site. This was characterized by edema and both perivascular and intervascular infiltration of polymorphonuclear and mononuclear cells. Grossly, the underside of the tumor was hemorrhagic and distinct from saline-inoculated tumors at this interval. Eight days after BCG injection, tumor cell nests were surrounded by fibrotic components of the dermis, and many tumor cells showed signs of degeneration. The tumor site regressed by day 15 and was generally fibrotic with some evidence of syncytial histiocytosis. No intact tumor cells could be distinguished, while there were numerous areas of focal necrosis.

The major histologic changes in the draining SDA lymph node after tumor excision and after saline or BCG intralesional injections are compared in table 1. Except for a progressive metastatic growth of tumor cells, no other marked alterations occurred in SDA lymph nodes after saline injection. At 25 days after saline injection, a greatly enlarged SDA lymph node was entirely metastatic, with some small portions of lymphoid components (fig. 4). The PA and contralateral lymph nodes, while they showed no metastases, did contain a degree of reticuloendothelial activity, best described as histiocytosis.

A unique feature of the SDA lymph nodes in the tumor-excision group was a marked hyperplastic germinal center reaction in the cortical area (fig. 5). This was a very prominent alteration of the cortex, implying a unique reaction to metastatic tumor cells not seen in the presence of a growing tumor, as in the saline-inoculated group.

The metastases in the subcapsular marginal sinus were more extensive 1 day after BCG, compared to the SDA nodes of saline-inoculated or tumor-excision guinea pigs (fig. 6). We assume that there was a greater influx of tumor cells or tumor emboli via the afferent lymphatics as a result of the acute inflammatory response and the vascular alterations at the tumor site. In acid-fast stained preparations, mycobacteria were detected in the marginal sinus; the organisms were associated with macrophages seen in the marginal sinuses and were never seen in direct contact with tumor cells. On the ultrastructural level, encapsulated organisms were detected intracellularly in occasional reticuloendothelial cells (fig. 7a).

At day 4 after BCG injection the architecture of the ipsilateral SDA lymph node was markedly altered (fig. 8). Tumor cell penetration into the cortex had destroyed the follicular configuration, and an absence of active germinal centers was noted. Noncaseous granulomas were observed throughout the cortex, bordering the metastatic rim of the node. Small numbers of mycobacteria were occasionally detected in these granulomas. Histologically the focal granulomas consisted of concentrations of histiocytes, and mitotic figures were common in these structures. The characteristic features of the histiocytes involved in granuloma formation are illustrated in figure 7b. Each cell has a large nucleus with the heterochromatin dispersed at its periphery in one or more discrete nuclei. The principal organelles of the voluminous cytoplasm are numerous small cisternae of rough-surfaced endoplasmic reticulum and large, electronlucent mitochondria. The intercellular space is filled with the interdigitation of the slender, fingerlike processes of the cytoplasm of these cells. In the subcapsular and medullary sinuses of the regional draining lymph nodes these histiocytes and lymphocytes induced degeneration, although not phagocytosis, of metastatic tumor cells. In the medullary sinuses of these nodes the histiocytes were frequently in close association with tumor cells, and some of the tumor cells showed definite signs of degeneration (fig. 7c, d; fig. 9).

Eight days after BCG injection (15 days after tumor cell injection) the architecture of the ipsilateral SDA lymph nodes consisted of coalesced granulomas occupying the major portion of the cortical and paracortical regions of the node. In some areas the granulomatous reaction had become generally infiltrated with polymorphonuclear cells. Residual tumor cells within these reaction centers showed signs of degeneration (fig. 10). There was a marked decrease in the number of tumor cells in these nodes. Granulomas but no tumor cells were observed in the ipsilateral axillary nodes.

At 25 days after intralesional BCG injection the ipsilateral SDA nodes were reduced in size from the previous interval (fig. 11), and a syncytial histiocytosis occupied most of the node (fig. 12). Distinct sinuses were rare, and areas of focal necrosis were seen throughout the node. Small but discrete regions of lymphoid components could still be observed.

Comparison of BCG With Inflammatory and Sensitizing Agents

We have also compared BCG-induced reactivity and the reactions induced by turpentine, vaccinia virus, and oxazolone in the interdermal tumor and the regional lymph node (*14*). Text-figure 1 shows the effects of various treatments on the rate of tumor growth. Between 8 and 20 days all treatments slightly increased papule size, compared to the saline-inoculated controls, as a result of the immediate inflammatory response at the site of sensitization. Twelve to 13 days after intratumor injection of BCG, the tumors began to regress and eventually disappeared. After the initial inflammatory response, the vaccinia virus-treated tumors grew at the same rate as the saline-injected controls. Both turpentine- and oxazolone-treated tumors grew faster than tumors of saline-inoculated controls. At day 55 the tumor mass in oxazolone- and turpentine-treated guinea pigs was about twice that of the control animals.

Table 1 summarizes the major changes in the regional lymph nodes during the first 25 days after treatment from these various agents. In the regional lymph nodes responding to intratumor injections of vaccinia virus and oxazolone, in contrast to the granulomatous reactivity of BCG-treated animals, there was extensive proliferation of cells

205

in the thymus-dependent region (paracortex) of the node (fig. 13). Macrophages laden with pigment were abundant in the medullary sinuses of these nodes, as well as in the nodes of turpentine-treated animals. The reaction observed in the lymph nodes of oxazolone- and vaccinia virus-treated animals was similar to that which accompanies the development of delayed-type hypersensitivity.

At 8 days after treatment with oxazolone and vaccinia virus, the hyperreactivity of the paracortex

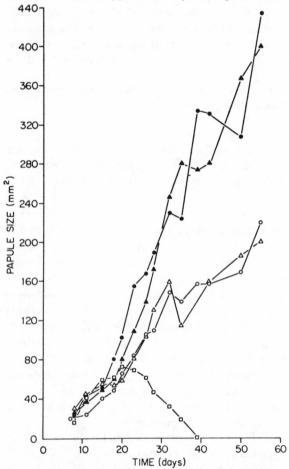

Text-figure 1.—Tumor growth calculated from mean papule size (r^2) after various treatments: O, saline (controls); □, BCG; △, vaccinia virus; ●, oxazolone; ▲, turpentine.

TABLE 1.—Major histologic changes in the draining lymph node following various treatments of intradermal tumor

Time after treatment (days)	Major histologic change	Treatment					
		Tumor excision	Saline	BCG	Vaccinia	Oxazolone	Turpentine
1	Tumor cells in marginal sinus	+	+	+	+	+	+
4	Tumor cells in marginal and medullary sinuses	+	+	+	+	+	+
	Granulomas in cortex and paracortex	−	−	++	−	−	−
	Histocytes and lymphocytes in medullary sinuses	−	−	++	−	−	−
	Active macrophages and lymphocytes in medullary sinuses	−	−	−	+	+	+
	Extensive proliferation of blast cells in cortical and paracortical regions	+	−	−	+	+	−
8	Tumor cells throughout node	+	+	+/−	+	+	+
	Coalesced granulomas	−	−	+	−	−	−
	Germinal centers	−	−	−	+	+	−
	Plasma cells	−	−	−	+	+	−
	Extensive proliferation of blast cells in cortical and paracortical regions	+	−	−	+	+	−
25	Metastatic lymph node	++	++	−	++	++	++
	Dilated, cystic sinuses	−	−	−	−	−	−
	Syncytial histiocytosis	−	−	+	−	−	−
	Extensive proliferation of blast cells in cortical and paracortical regions	+	−	−	−	−	−

207

of the node was still present, with active germinal centers in the cortex and plasma cells in the medullary sinuses. No such reactivity was observed in the nodes draining turpentine-inoculated tumor sites.

At 25 days after treatment, the draining regional lymph nodes in the turpentine-, oxazolone-, and vaccinia virus-treated guinea pigs were metastatic, possessing dilated fluid-filled spaces. In the nodes draining oxazolone- and vaccinia virus-treated tumors, occasional active germinal centers could still be observed, with large areas of polymorphonuclear cell abscesses. The reaction of the regional lymph nodes at 25 days in the oxazolone- and vaccinia virus-treated animals was in marked contrast to the tumor-free regional nodes of BCG-treated tumors.

DISCUSSION

There are three major components of the immune system: humoral antibody, cytotoxic lymphocytes, and reticuloendothelial cells such as mononuclear cells, histiocytes, and macrophages. As pointed out by Gorer (15), the effectiveness of these components is not equal at all sites and their individual or combined efficiency may be limited by anatomical factors. In a discussion of the limitations of these three components of the immune system in host-tumor interactions, Alexander (16) pointed out that the "success of antigenic tumor occurs for the same reasons that permit infectious diseases to establish themselves and to persist in immunologically competent hosts." That is, survival of tubercle bacilli in the heart valve is likened to the success of an antigenic tumor. Both occur because anatomic factors limit the full expression of the effector arms of the immune system. Accepting this, there is increasing evidence of a further limitation of the immune system in the host-tumor interaction, which is that two effector components of the immune system interact competitively or antagonistically. Antibody specific to tumor transplantation antigen has been shown *in vitro* to prevent sensitized lymphocytes from being cytotoxic to tumor cells (17); and it has been suggested that tumor antigen-anti-

208

body complexes may neutralize the activity of cytotoxic lymphocytes by binding to surface receptor sites (18).

In general, less attention has been devoted to the reticuloendothelial component and its activity in host-tumor interaction, probably because it does not demonstrate the degree of immunologic specificity expressed by antibody or sensitized lymphocytes. The major limitation of this effector arm of the immune system is cell concentration at the primary or disseminated tumor sites. Alexander (26) demonstrated that peritoneal "macrophages" isolated from animals immunized against a specific tumor or from animals with progressively growing tumors can destroy tumor cells in vitro. Phagocytosis was not involved in this cytotoxic reaction. The paradox here is that the tumor grows progressively in an animal that has sufficient number of peritoneal mononuclear cells to destroy it. Zbar et al. (19) elucidated this point in studies that demonstrated the failure of a transplanted guinea pig hepatocarcinoma to survive at a skin site in which erythema and induration had been induced by prior injection of a "macrophage-rich fraction" of peritoneal cells. Thus a critical concentration of peritoneal cells was capable of killing the tumor by virtue of a nonspecific response.

The effective antitumor reaction in BCG-treated animals is a nonspecific granulomatous reaction, characterized by an intense proliferation of stromal reticuloendothelial components and histiocytes. In contrast, lymphoproliferative cellular reactions characteristic of developing delayed-type hypersensitivity and nonspecific inflammatory reaction do not have detrimental effects on the tumor. It is apparent from the comparison of BCG-treated normal and BCG-treated tumor-bearing guinea pigs that the qualitative and quantitative characteristics of the granulomatous reaction, both at the tumor site and in draining lymph nodes, is only a function of a specific immunologic reaction provoked by the microorganism. Granulomatous inflammation is generally defined as the reticuloendothelial cell response to tissue injury, mediated by

209

a poorly soluble substance (11). It may be characterized as a foreign-body response as to a colloidal substance, generally involving a simple phagocytic process, or as a more intense proliferative reaction, involving primarily the stromal reticuloendothelial components and/or histiocytes. The granulomatous reaction is characteristic of the BCG-tumor system in the present study.

The question of immunologic specificity, or of developed immunity in the BCG granulomatous reaction in a syngeneic tumor system, is difficult to evaluate at present. It has been established that the BCG-mediated regression of transplantable syngeneic hepatocarcinoma and elimination of regional lymph node metastases is a two-step process (5). The first step is immunologically specific for BCG antigen. We have further data to support this analysis, based on the inability of BCG to induce tumor regression in animals made immunologically incompetent by antilymphocyte therapy (unpublished data). The second step, which is effective in destroying tumor cells, is probably immunologically nonspecific. There is evidence, however, that during tumor regression specific tumor immunity is developed, mediated by lymphocytes as well as detectable antitumor-specific antibody. It has been demonstrated that the syngeneic hepatocarcinomas used in the present study are rejected when they are reintroduced into guinea pigs that have recovered from tumor cell-BCG granulomatous reaction (20). These results suggest that lymphocyte sensitization does occur during the granulomatous reaction, and based on studies by Olson et al. (21), which demonstrate that regional lymph nodes draining BCG sensitization sites are anergic, one would have to assume that the developing lymphocyte sensitization during a BCG granulomatous response probably occurs systemically in peripheral lymphatic tissue as well as in the draining lymph nodes.

It is important that we consider the mechanism of BCG-induced tumor regression and elimination of regional lymph node metastases as a nonspecific reaction mediated by the physiologically altered and possibly detrimental environment created by

210

the granulomatous reaction at the tumor site in the draining lymph node. Constriction of postcapillary venules has been described in lymph nodes reacting to certain delayed hypersensitivity antigens (21, 22). There is good reason to believe that this condition is also created by BCG in the node, causing infarction in the affected areas, and that as a result tumor cells which normally grow well in draining lymph nodes (as seen in the saline-inoculated and tumor-excision animals) find the environment of a granulomatous reaction detrimental to growth. While this may account for part of the destruction of the metastatic growth, it still does not completely explain the subtle histiocyte-tumor cell interactions in the lymph node sinuses, where there are obvious signs of tumor cell degeneration. This response of histiocytes and tumor cells is reminiscent of the "activated" histiocyte-tumor cell interaction described by others in *in vitro* as well as *in vivo* systems (23–26). The cytopathic mechanism by which such "activated" histiocytes destroy tumor cells is not completely understood; however, it does not appear to be simply a phagocytic process. Furthermore, there is at present little or no evidence to support the contention that an immunologically specific histiocyte hypersensitivity to the tumor is developed. Also, the effectiveness of the granulomatous reaction in completely eliminating tumor and metastases is most certainly based on the propensity of this tumor system to metastasize to the lymph nodes via the afferent lymphatic, as is the case for many tumors in man, rather than to other sites via the bloodstream. This is a critical aspect of the system, since the early inflammatory reaction enhances general dissemination of tumor cells, a consequence of vascular alterations of the primary transplantation site.

It might be reasonable at this time to consider that a natural example of such a beneficial host-tumor interaction is the prognostically favorable reaction of draining lymph nodes to a prolonged exposure to neoplasia, such as carcinoma of the breast and stomach in man, originally described as "syncitial" and "sinus histiocytosis" by Black and

Speer (27). At present we are prone to make a histopathologic correlation between the general granulomatous reaction induced by BCG and syncytial histiocytosis in man.

In the light of the demonstrated success of intralesional injection of BCG in causing regression of transplanted syngeneic tumors and eliminating regional lymph node metastases, a stronger consideration should be made of the use of induced granulomatous reactivity as primary treatment as well as an adjunct of any immunotherapeutic or chemotherapeutic model for the treatment of tumors. It is possible that tumor growth normally precedes the development of specific cell-mediated immunity to a degree which constantly favors the tumor system. The induction of a granulomatous reaction at the tumor site and in the regional node during the early stages of metastasis would confine and destroy the major mass of tumor, at the same time releasing processed tumor antigen. Thereby, the major portion of the tumor would be destroyed presumably with release of tumor antigen as a result of concentration of histiocytes, allowing for the development of a systemic cell-mediated immunity capable of reaching and eliminating any tumor cells that by-passed or escaped the granulomatous reaction.

The major difference between tumor excision and the induced granulomatous reaction is the quantitative difference in the systemic release of processed tumor antigen, and thus in the degree of specific cell-mediated immunity. Furthermore, an organism such as BCG can distribute its activation capability both at the tumor site and in the regional and perhaps other peripheral nodes, the major location of tumor cells during the early intervals of the response. That this is important is seen in the fact that when BCG is injected into tumors later than 7 days after transplantation, when the tumor has increased in size and metastasis has become more widespread and disseminated, it is considerably less effective (20). The experiments described and the explanation given here should provide a basis for further experimental studies of the advantages

212

of this tumor-killing mechanism in conjunction with development of specific tumor immunity.

REFERENCES

(1) RAPP HJ, CHURCHILL WH JR, KRONMAN BS, et al: Antigenicity of a new diethylnitrosamine-induced transplantable guinea pig hepatoma: Pathology and formation of ascites variant. J Natl Cancer Inst 41: 1–7, 1968

(2) KRONMAN B, WEPSIC HT, CHURCHILL WH JR, et al: Immunotherapy of cancer: An experimental model in syngeneic guinea pigs. Science 168:257–259, 1970

(3) ZBAR B, TANAKA T: Immunotherapy of cancer: Regression of tumors after intralesional injection of Mycobacterium bovis. Science 172:271–273, 1971

(4) BERNSTEIN ID, RAPP HJ: Impaired cellular immunity in tumor-bearing animals: A nonspecific mononuclear cell deficiency. Fed Proc 30:245, 1971

(5) ZBAR B, WEPSIC HT, BORSOS T, et al: Tumor-graft rejection in syngeneic guinea pigs: Evidence for a two-step mechanism. J Natl Cancer Inst 44:475–481, 1970

(6) SPECTOR WG: Histology of allergic inflammation. Br Med Bull 23:35–38, 1967

(7) KOSUNEN TU, WAKSMAN BH, SAMUELSON IK: Radioautographic study of cellular mechanisms in delayed hypersensitivity. J Neuropathol Exp Neurol 22:367–380, 1963

(8) VOLKMAN A, GOWANS JL: The production of macrophages in the rat. Br J Exp Pathol 46:50–61, 1965

(9) ———: The origin of macrophages from bone marrow in the rat. Br J Exp Pathol 46:62–70, 1965

(10) HANNA MG JR, ZBAR B, RAPP HJ: Histopathology of tumor regression following intralesional injection of Mycobacterium bovis (BCG). I. Tumor growth and metastasis. J Natl Cancer Inst 48:1441–1455, 1972

(11) EPSTEIN WL: Granulomatous hypersensitivity. Progr Allergy 11:36–88, 1967

(12) GAAFAR SM, TURK JL: Granuloma formation in lymph nodes. J Pathol 100:9–20, 1970

(13) DANNENBERG AM JR: Cellular hypersensitivity and cellular immunity in the pathogenesis of tuberculosis: Specificity, systemic and local nature, and associated macrophage enzymes. Bacteriol Rev 32:85–102, 1968

(14) HANNA MG JR, ZBAR B, RAPP JH: Histopathology of tumor regression following intralesional injection of Mycobacterium bovis (BCG). II. Comparative effects of vaccinia virus, oxazolone, and turpentine. J Natl Cancer Inst 48:1697–1707, 1972

(15) GORER PA: The antigenic structure of tumors. Adv Immunol 1:345–393, 1961

(16) ALEXANDER P: Factors contributing to the "success" of antigen tumors. *In* Morphologic and Functional Aspects of Immunity (Lindahl-Kiessling K, Alm G, Hanna MG Jr., eds.). New York, Plenum, 1971, pp 567–574

(17) HELLSTRÖM I, HELLSTRÖM KE: Studies on cellular immunity and its serum mediated inhibition on Moloney-virus-induced mouse sarcomas. Int J Cancer 4:587–600, 1969

(18) SJÖGREN HO, HELLSTRÖM I, BANSAL SC, et al: Suggestive evidence that the "blocking antibodies" of tumor-bearing individuals may be antigen-antibody complexes. Proc Natl Acad Sci USA 68:1372–1375, 1971

(19) ZBAR B, BERNSTEIN ID, RAPP HJ: Suppression of tumor growth by peritoneal exudate macrophages from unimmunized strain 2 guinea pigs. Proc Am Assoc Cancer Res 11:87, 1970

(20) ZBAR B, BERNSTEIN ID, BARTLETT GL, et al: Immunotherapy of cancer: Regression of intradermal tumors and prevention of growth of lymph node metastases after intralesional injection of living *Mycobacterium bovis* (bacillus Calmette-Guérin). J Natl Cancer Inst 49:119–130, 1972

(21) OLSON IA, HUNT AC, VERRIER-JONES J: Competition between two delayed hypersensitivity antigens for the same draining lymph-node: The histiocytic response compared with sinus histiocytosis. J Pathol 103:107–111, 1971

(22) DE SOUSA MA, PARROTT D: Induction and recall in contact sensitivity. Changes in skin and draining lymph nodes of intact and thymectomized mice. J Exp Med 130:671–690, 1969

(23) GORER PA: Some recent work on tumor immunity. Adv Cancer Res 4:149–156, 1956

(24) AMOS DB: The use of simplified systems as an aid to the interpretation of mechanisms of graft rejection. Progr Allergy 6:468–538, 1962

(25) GERSHON RK, CARTER RL, LANE NJ: Studies on homotransplantable lymphomas in hamsters. IV. Observations on macrophages in the expression of tumor immunity. Am J Pathol 51:1111–1133, 1967

(26) ALEXANDER P, EVANS R: Endotoxin and double stranded RNA render macrophages cytotoxic. Nature [New Biol] (Lond) 232:76–78, 1971

(27) BLACK MM, SPEER FD: Sinus histiocytosis of lymph nodes in cancer. Surg Gynecol Obstet 106:163–175, 1958

214

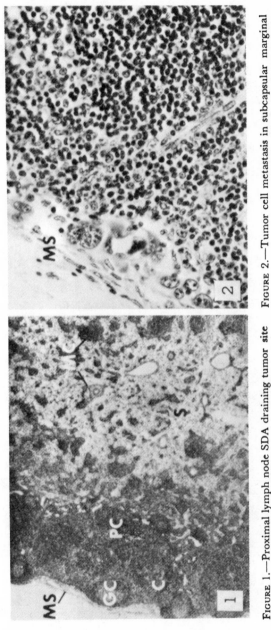

FIGURE 1.—Proximal lymph node SDA draining tumor site 4 days after tumor cell injection. MS = marginal sinus; GC = germinal center; C = cortex; PC = paracortex; S = medullary sinuses; MC = medullary cords. Hematoxylin and eosin. × 30

FIGURE 2.—Tumor cell metastasis in subcapsular marginal sinus (MS) of SDA lymph node 7 days after transplantation. Hematoxylin and eosin. × 300

215

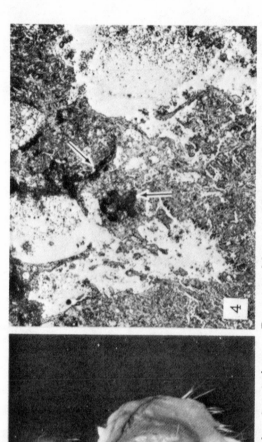

FIGURE 4.—Metastatic SDA lymph node after intratumor saline injection. *Note* residual lymphatic tissue (*arrows*) and cystic condition of node. Hematoxylin and eosin. × 30

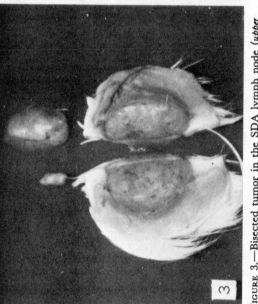

FIGURE 3.—Bisected tumor in the SDA lymph node (*upper right*) and contralateral lymph node (*upper left*) 25 days after saline injection.

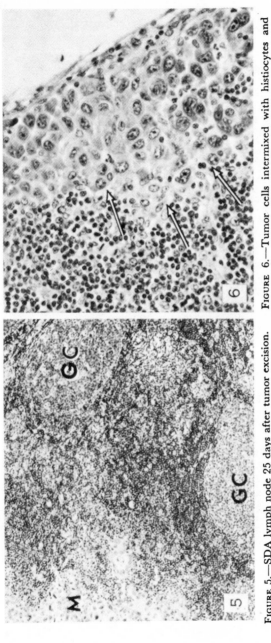

Figure 5.—SDA lymph node 25 days after tumor excision. *Note* hyperplastic germinal centers (GC) and extensive metastasis (M). Hematoxylin and eosin. × 125

Figure 6.—Tumor cells intermixed with histiocytes and macrophages (*arrows*) in the marginal sinus of the SDA lymph node of a BCG-inoculated tumor-bearing guinea pig 1 day after BCG (8 days after tumor transplantation). Hematoxylin and eosin. × 300

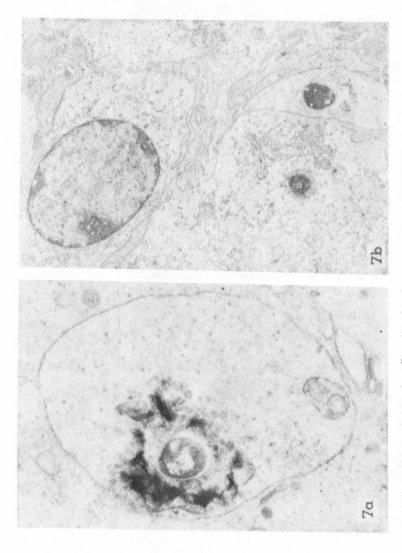

FIGURE 7.—Anatomy of stimulation of a cell-mediated anti-tumor response. *a*) BCG organism, cut in cross section, within a phagosome of a histiocyte in lymph node draining tumor site. × 41,000 *b*) Interdigitating histiocytes forming a "syncytial" granuloma in draining lymph node after stimulation with BCG. × 5,700

218

c) Three histiocytes and a lymphocyte in contact with a degenerating metastatic tumor cell in subcapsular sinus of lymph node draining tumor site 8 days after stimulation with BCG. × 5,500 d) Configuration suggestive of fusion of plasmalemmae of histiocyte (H) and tumor cell (T). × 24,000

219

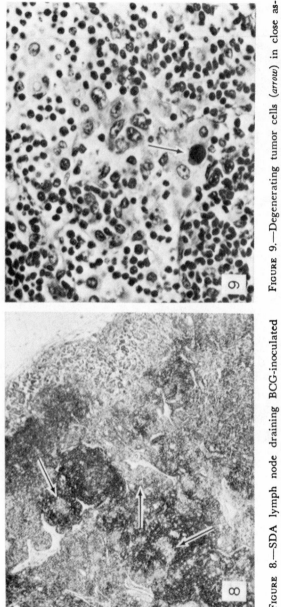

FIGURE 8.—SDA lymph node draining BCG-inoculated tumor 4 days after BCG injection. *Note* extensive metastasis (*upper right*), histiocyte-infiltrated medullary sinus (*lower left*), and granulomas (*arrows*). Hematoxylin and eosin. × 30

FIGURE 9.—Degenerating tumor cells (*arrow*) in close association with sinusoid histiocytes. SDA lymph node 4 days after intratumor BCG injection. Hematoxylin and eosin. × 300

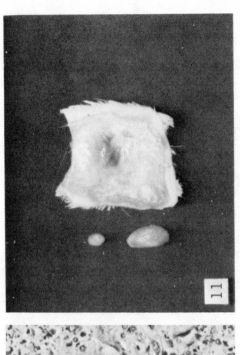

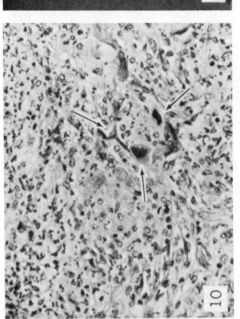

Figure 10.—Degenerating tumor cells (*arrows*) trapped in granulomatous reaction centers of SDA lymph nodes 8 days after intratumor BCG injection. Hematoxylin and eosin. × 300

Figure 11.—Remnant of tumor site 25 days after BCG injection. SDA lymph node (*bottom left*) and contralateral lymph node (*top left*).

221

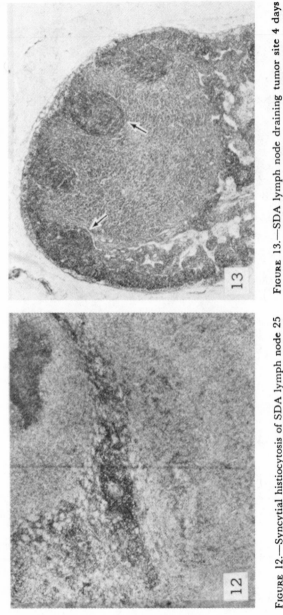

FIGURE 13.—SDA lymph node draining tumor site 4 days after external application of oxazolone. *Note* distinct follicles in cortex (*arrows*) and the distended paracortex. Hematoxylin and eosin. X 30

FIGURE 12.—Syncytial histiocytosis of SDA lymph node 25 days after intratumor BCG injection. *Note* residual lymphoid component (*center*) and focal necrotic mass (*upper right*). Hematoxylin and eosin. X 30

Fetal Thymic Transplant in Patients With Hodgkin's Disease

Roberto Marcolongo and Nicola Di Paolo

Five patients with Hodgkin's disease were treated by transplantation of fetal thymic tissue. Clinical and immunologic studies, carried out for over 5 mo thereafter, revealed a prompt improvement in previously defective cellular immune functions, including a significant rise of absolute lymphocytes in the peripheral blood and a nor-malization of tuberculin skin sensitivity and of the response of peripheral blood lymphocytes to phytohemagglutinin. It is suggested that fetal thymic transplant into patients with Hodgkin's disease appears at present the best tool of improving their immunologic deficiency.

THERE HAVE BEEN a number of observations that suggest severe impairment of the peripheral lymphoid function in Hodgkin's disease.[1] These are the depression of delayed hypersensitivity,[2] the abnormal response from patients with Hodgkin's disease to phytohemagglutinin (PHA) in vitro[3] in the face of essentially normal antibody formation,[4] and the recovery of skin allergy during disease remission.[1] Various authors have reported data indicating a failure of delayed sensitivity reactions, in part dependent on the duration of the disease;[1] decreased cutaneous reactions are characteristic of Hodgkin's disease at all times[5] but are most marked when the disease is active and widespread.[6,7] This immunologic deficiency is a feature of early stages of Hodgkin's disease, but the depression of delayed hypersensitivity becomes more profound as the disease becomes advanced and more generalized.[1,5,8] Lamb et al.[9] emphasized that, while patients with cancer, leukemia, and non-Hodgkin's lymphoma frequently are anergic when in poor clinical condition, those patients with Hodgkin's are anergic even though their clinical status is good. However, several authors have shown that the severity of the defect in cellular immune mechanisms varies with the clinical activity of Hodgkin's disease and that anergic patients may regain a positive skin test

223

response after successful treatment.[1,9-13] In a study of 50 untreated patients, the abnormalities characteristically associated with Hodgin's disease were seen in the later and more active stages.[14]

Recent data on the histopathology and immunology of postneonatal thymectomized animals[15,16] raised the possibility that Hodgkin's disease might be considered as a syndrome of hypothymism. Svet-Moldavsky[17] suggested that the pathogenesis of Hodgkin's disease is based on a definite hypothymic-hypolymphocytic syndrome characterized by depletion and quantitative deficiency of the lymphocytes of lymphoid organs, by lymphopenia in the peripheral blood, by enhanced proliferation of reticular and immature plasma cells, and by loss of immunologic responses of the delayed type with retained capacity for antibody production. The results obtained by thymus transplants in DiGeorge's syndrome[18-20] prompted us to attempt to reconstitute the immunologic function by thymic transplantation in patients with Hodgkin's disease.

This report describes the development of immunologic function in a series of patients with Hodgkin's disease after the implantation of fetal thymic tissue.

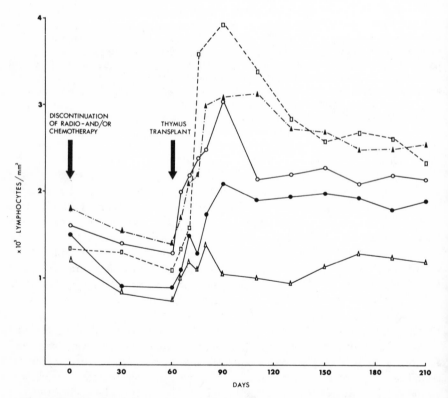

Fig. 1. Absolute lymphocyte counts (cells/cu mm) of peripheral blood in patients with Hodgkin's disease before and periodically after thymus grafts. Open triangles, case 1; open squares, case 2; black circles, case 3; black triangles, case 4; open circles, case 5.

Table 1. Absolute Lymphocyte Counts* in Patients With Hodgkin's Disease Before and Following Implantation of Fetal Thymus

Cases	Stage	At End of Radio— and/or Chemotherapy Treatment	Before Implantation	4-10 Days After Implantation	Maximal Lymphocyte Number Increase 20-30 Days After Implantation	5 Mo After Implantation
1	IV A	1200 ± 115	750 ± 50	1200 ± 220	1400 ± 170	1200 ± 170
2	III B	1350 ± 80	1100 ± 110	1600 ± 140	3950 ± 240	2350 ± 220
3	III A	1450 ± 105	900 ± 80	1500 ± 110	2100 ± 130	1900 ± 110
4	III A	1800 ± 195	1400 ± 150	2100 ± 130	3150 ± 370	2550 ± 230
5	III B	1600 ± 180	1250 ± 280	2200 ± 280	3050 ± 190	2150 ± 150

*Absolute lymphocyte counts, cells/cu mm.

MATERIALS AND METHODS

We have studied five patients with Hodgkin's disease. To be included in the study, patients were required to have histologically verified disease that appeared to be progressive and that could be followed by serial objective measurements. All subjects were in an advanced stage of the disease (Stage III and IV [21] and had been previously treated for several months with radiotherapy or cyclic low-dose combination chemotherapy of cyclophosphamide, vincristine or methylhydrazine, and corticosteroids. Treatment was not continual, but our patients were allowed to relapse and then were retreated periodically.[22] At the time of the study, all the patients were in a relapsing stage of the disease and had had no treatment for about 2 mo prior to the study. Thymus glands from 25 to 32-wk-old fetuses that died after premature births were implanted within 4–8 hr of removal under the fascia of the rectus abdominis muscle. During the period from removal to implantation, the thymus was kept in tissue culture medium 199 at +4°C. Complete blood counts and immunologic studies, consisting of tuberculin skin tests and in vitro studies of lymphocyte function, were carried out periodically after thymic implantation. Tuberculin (purified protein derivative, PPD) was injected intradermally on the forearm in 0.1 ml sterile saline solution, and the reaction was read 12, 24, and 48 hr later; only erythema and induration greater than 5 mm in diameter were considered to be unequivocally positive. Peripheral blood leukocytes were cultured by standard methods[23] at concentrations of approximately 1 × 10^6 mononuclear cells/ml in a medium consisting of 80% TC 199 and 20% autologous plasma; phytohemagglutinin (PHA, Difco) was added to cultures at a concentration of 10 μg/ml. Cultures were incubated for 72 hr. After this period the cells were harvested, and smears were made and stained with May-Grünwald-Giemsa stain.

RESULTS

Four to 10 days after the transplant, a significative rise of lymphocytes took place in all five patients, and during the following five mo normal lymphocyte counts were recorded (Fig. 1 and Table 1). For comparison, Fig. 2 and Table 2 give lymphocyte counts in four nontransplanted Hodgkin's patients who were followed during a period of clinical remission induced by cyclic chemotherapy equivalent to that of the transplanted patients. By 2 wk after implantation of fetal thymus, our patients showed a normal delayed hypersensitivity to tuberculin and this was maintained (Table 3). The response of the peripheral lymphocytes to PHA was nearly completely normal when evaluated 15–20 days after the transplant and remained so (Table 4). Our patients showed only a partial recovery from the clinical manifestations of

Table 2. Absolute Lymphocyte Counts* in a Group of Patients With Hodgkin's Disease During a Period of Clinical Remission Induced by Cyclic Chemotherapy

Cases	Stage	At End of Chemotherapy Treatment	After 1 Mo	After 2 Mo	After 3 Mo	After 4 Mo	After 5 Mo	After 6 Mo	After 7 Mo
1	II A	2000 ± 210	2175 ± 150	2100 ± 75	1820 ± 96	1800 ± 74	2100 ± 108	2200 ± 104	2100 ± 88
2	II A	1830 ± 98	1600 ± 135	1800 ± 82	1900 ± 102	2000 ± 116	2000 ± 80	1800 ± 70	2000 ± 106
3	II B	1500 ± 105	1450 ± 150	1700 ± 100	1600 ± 124	1750 ± 120	1600 ± 90	1500 ± 100	1700 ± 88
4	III A	1150 ± 85	1380 ± 118	1500 ± 112	1400 ± 130	1300 ± 68	1200 ± 45	1570 ± 72	1600 ± 120

*Absolute lymphocyte counts, cells/cu mm.

Table 3. Skin Test Response in Patients With Hodgkin's Disease Before
and Following Implantation of Fetal Thymus

Cases	Stage	Before Implantation	15 Days After Implantation	3 Mo After Implantation	5 Mo After Implantation
1	IV A	0	±	+	+
2	III B	0	+	+	+
3	III A	0	+	+	+
4	III A	0	2+	2+	+
5	III B	0	+	+	+

Scoring skin tests: 0–5 mm induration and erythema, ±; 5–10 mm induration and erythema, +; > 10 mm induration and erythema, 2+; 0, no induration and erythema.

Hodgkin's disease. It is known that an optimum symptomatic result can be established when inflammation and other specific symptoms of Hodgkin's disease are completely suppressed.[24] To obtain a complete remission, the patient's subjective complaints, physical examination, performance status, and laboratory and radiologic data must return to normal.[25,26] Our patients, however, had marked but not complete remission of lymphadenopathy and organomegaly and improvement in subjective response and thus were considered to have a partial remission (Table 4 and Fig. 2).[26] In our patients the improvement was limited to a diminution of lymph nodes size and to amelioration of the general symptomatology, as well as regression of objective findings, such as fever, and a progressive but significant decrease of sedimentation rate. None of the patients appeared to have signs of graft-vs-host reactions during the 5 mo that they were followed after the fetal thymus was implanted. During this time the newly acquired immunologic competence persisted, and their clinical condition was satisfactory. Histologic studies of the survival of the transplanted thymus were not obtained, since it would have required additional surgery. Some authors,[27,28] however, have presented evidence that implanted fetal thymus fragments are capable of long-term survival when implanted in muscle. In several cases the implants have been studied at necroscopy, and at least some of the pieces have been found to be viable, and the histology of the thymus was well preserved.

DISCUSSION

The immunologic defects observed in our patients before thymic graft may have arisen as a result of cytotoxic drugs or x-ray therapy, for these may

Table 4. Transformation of Lymphocytes From Patients With Hodgkin's Disease Before and Following Implantation of Fetal Thymus (Per Cent Lymphocyte Responsiveness to PHA)

Cases	Stage	Before Implantation	15-20 Days After Implantation	3 Mo After Implantation	5 Mo After Implantation
1	IV A	12	38	42	35
2	III B	42	66	62	65
3	III A	20	57	61	58
4	III A	39	70	67	63
5	III B	35	62	72	68

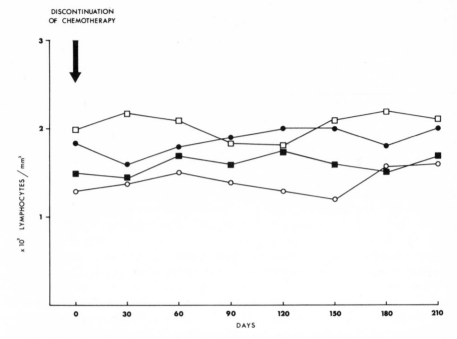

Fig. 2. Absolute lymphocyte counts (cells/cu mm) of peripheral blood in a group of patients with Hodgkin's disease during a period of clinical remission induced by cyclic chemotherapy.

cause cellular damage.[29] Thus the question arises of whether the improvement in immunologic responsiveness and the rise in blood lymphocytes was due to the withdrawal of immunosuppressive chemotherapy or to the implantation of thymus tissue. Radiotherapy and most chemotherapeutic agents are known to have immunosuppressive effects,[30-32] so that it is necessary to distinguish these effects from those attributable to Hodgkin's disease. It seems unlikely that the immune deficiency was the result of previous x-ray, cytotoxic drugs, or steroid treatment. Sokal and Primikirios[5] emphasized that the doses of alkylating agents or x-ray necessary to suppress immunity are substantially greater than those used clinically in the treatment of Hodgkin's disease or other lymphomas. On the other hand, several authors have observed that many patients recovered normal tuberculin sensitivity or skin reactivity against other antigens shortly after remission was induced by x-ray or chemotherapy.[5,25] Schneider[33] and Migueres et al.[34] studied the effect of different types of chemotherapeutic agents on the development of delayed hypersensitivity reactions in patients with Hodgkin's disease, lymphomas, and lung cancer. During the course of therapy, some positive reactions became negative and the converse was also observed, some negative reactions became positive. In still others there was no change. These authors demonstrated, however, that the continuous administration of drugs led more frequently to positive reactions becoming negative than was seen with discontinuous or cyclic therapy. De Vita et al.[25] observed that most patients with Hodgkin's disease were anergic before therapy, and reversion of skin tests

228

to positive was common in those tested in remission. Elves et al.[29] reported that some of their patients with Hodgkin's disease who had a normal lymphocyte transformation had received nitrogen mustard therapy for some months before study. Astaldi et al.[35] observed that cultures from Hodgkin's patients made before treatment showed minimal transformation, but after x-ray therapy normal numbers of blasts were present in cultures. Trubowitz et al.[36] demonstrated an improvement in the capacity of lymphocytes to transform as symptoms ameliorated during remission of Hodgkin's disease. Goldman et al.[6] observed that three of four patients with active Stage III or IV Hodgkin's and nodular sclerosis had normal lymphocyte responsiveness to PHA even when undergoing chemotherapy. Tansini et al.[37] studied the lymphocyte response to PHA in patients with neoplastic diseases before and after cytotoxic treatment. They did not find significant changes when using combinations of chemotherapeutic drugs for long-term periods; both discontinuous and cyclic chemotherapy was used. These findings suggest that treatment with immunosuppressive drugs does not impair the ability to recover responsiveness to delayed hypersensitivity antigens, particularly when chemotherapy is discontinuous or interrupted for a significant period, as in our patients.

After implantation of thymus tissue our patients regained their immunologic competence, suggesting that, as in DiGeorge's syndrome, the immunologic defect in Hodgkin's disease may lie in the effector portion of the immune response. Indeed, the observations on the thymus implants in DiGeorge's syndrome showed that the major part at least of the repopulation of peripheral lymphoid tissues was from host rather than from donor cells. The chromosomal studies of Cleveland et al.[19] and August et al.[18] proved that the cells that responded normally in vitro to PHA stimuli after the graft were derived from the patients rather than from the grafted fetal thymus. Many arguments suggest that these cells may originate in the bone marrow.[38] It is probable that the transplanted thymus confers on the host lymphocytes the capacity to respond, rather than serving as the source of the dividing cells. There is presently no indication whether thymus implanted under these circumstances serves as a source of so-called thymus hormone[38] or whether its reticular-epithelial elements directly influence the patient's lymphoid cells. Svet-Moldavsky[17] underlined that the concept of the syndrome of hypothymism in Hodgkin's disease is not equivalent to hypofunction or lack of function of the thymus. The syndrome may depend on hypofunction of the thymus, while at the same time developing from a blocking of the transmission of hormonal or other thymus effects to the effector systems at different levels. Indeed, the syndrome does not necessarily imply a morphologic involvement of the thymus in the process. It remains completely unclear, however, how the immunologic deficiency is related to the pathogenesis of Hodgkin's disease. The specific question is what relationship, if any, there is among conditions with thymic aplasia (as in DiGeorge's syndrome), the thymectomy-wasting syndrome, and Hodgkin's disease. The similarity with wasting disease of lymphoid origin with associated immunologic impairment is suggestive. Lymphoid depletion and the susceptibility to secondary infections offer further analogies. Thymic aplasia and the thymectomy-wasting syndrome, however, would not seem to account for localized Hodkin's disease and for the histologic picture, fever and leukocytosis of disseminated disease. Furthermore, in neonatally thymectomized animals, in contrast to the Hodgkin's patients, lymphocyte depletion occurs early and depression of antibody formation may be associated with the depression of delayed hypersensitivity.[1]

Our results encourage us to suggest that transplantation of thymus tissue should be further evaluated in patients with Hodgkin's disease as a method for successful reconstitution of immunologic function. The duration of the clinical and immunologic improvement is at present unknown, and it remains to be demonstrated whether the immunologic reconstitution obtained in our cases signifies a more favorable prognosis. It must be also emphasized that the small sample size of the present study does not permit any definitive conclusion. Longer-term studies are required to evaluate this finding. However, even if the thymus transplant procedure does not completely cure Hodgkin's patients, it should result in a marked improvement of many phenomena associated with the state of functional hypothymism.

These facts indicate that, until purified thymus hormone or cellular immunity mediators become available, implants of fetal thymus into patients with Hodgkin's disease offer at present the best possibility to ameliorate their serious immunologic deficiency.

REFERENCES

1. Molander DW, Pack GT: Hodgkin's Disease. Springfield, Ill., Thomas, 1968, p 64

2. Aisenberg AC: Manifestations of immunologic unresponsiveness in Hodgkin's disease. Cancer Res 26:1152, 1966

3. Hersh EM, Oppenheim JJ: Impaired in vitro lymphocyte transformation in Hodgkin's disease. N Engl J Med 273:1006, 1965

4. Aisenberg AC, Leskowitz S: Antibody formation in Hodgkin's disease. N Engl J Med 268:1269, 1963

5. Sokal JE, Primikirios N: The delayed skin test response in Hodgkin's disease and lymphosarcoma. Cancer 14:597, 1961

6. Goldman JM, Hobbs JR: The immunoglobulins in Hodgkin's disease. Immunology 13:421, 1967

7. Nagel GA: Immunosuppression: ein paraneoplastisches Syndrom. Schweiz Med Wochenschr 101:470, 1971

8. Sokal JE: Discussion on: Manifestations of immunological unresponsiveness in Hodgkin's disease. Cancer Res 26:1161, 1966

9. Lamb D, Pilney F, Kelly WD, Good RA: A comparative study of the incidence of anergy in patients with carcinoma, leukemia, Hodgkin's disease and other lymphomas. J. Immunol 89:555, 1962

10. Aisenberg AC: Studies on delayed hypersensitivity in Hodgkin's disease. J Clin Invest 41:1964, 1962

11. Chase MW: Delayed-type hypersensitivity and the immunology of Hodgkin's disease, with a parallel examination of sarcoidosis. Cancer Res 26:1097, 1966

12. Dubin IN: Poverty of immunological mechanism in patients with Hodgkin's disease. Ann Intern Med 27:898, 1967

13. Sokal JE, August CW: Response to BCG vaccination and survival in advanced Hodgkin's disease. Cancer 24:128, 1969

14. Brown RS, Haynes HA, Foley HT, Godwin HA, Berard CW, Carbone PP: Hodgkin's disease. Immunologic, clinical, and histologic features of 50 untreated patients. Ann Intern Med 67:291, 1967

15. Miller JFAP: Effect of neonatal thymectomy on the immunological responsiveness of the mouse. Proc R Soc Lond [Biol] 156:415, 1962

16. Waksman BH, Arnason BG, Jankovic, BD: Role of the thymus in immune reactions in rats. J Exp Med 116:159, 1962

17. Svet-Moldavsky GJ: Is Hodgkin's disease a syndrome of hypothymism? Nature (Lond) 209:932, 1966

18. August CS, Rosen FS, Filler, RM, Janeway CA, Markowski B, Kay HEM: Implantation of a foetal thymus, restoring immunological competence in a patient with thymic aplasia (Di George's syndrome). Lancet 2:1210, 1968

19. Cleveland W.W., Fogel BJ, Brown WT, Kay HEM: Foetal thymic transplant in a case of Di George's syndrome. Lancet 2:1211, 1968

20. August CS, Levey RH, Berkel AI, Rosen FS, Kay HEM: Establishment of immunological competence in a child with congenital thymic aplasia by a graft of fetal thymus. Lancet 1:1080, 1970

21. Rosenberg SA: Report of the committee on the staging of Hodgkin's disease. Cancer Res 26:1310, 1966

22. Carbone PP, Spurr C: Management of patients with malignant lymphoma. A comparative study with cyclophosphamide and vinca alkaloids. Cancer Res 28:811, 1968

23. Moorehead PS, Nowell PC, Mellman, WS, Battips, DM, Hungerford DA: Chromosome preparation of leukocytes cultured from human peripheral blood. Exp Cell Res 20:613, 1960

24. Anglesio E: The Treatment of Hodgkin's Disease. Berlin, New York, Springer-Verlag, 1969, p 50

25. De Vita VT, Serpick AA, Carbone PP: Combination chemotherapy in the treatment of advanced Hodgkin's disease. Ann Intern Med 73:881, 1970

26. Bagley CM, De Vita, VT, Berard CW, Canellos GP: Advanced lymphosarcoma: Intensive cyclical combination chemotherapy with cyclophosphamide, vincristine, and prednisone. Ann Intern Med 76:227, 1972

27. Gitlin D, Rosen FS, Janeway CA: The thymus and other lymphoid tissues in congenital agammaglobulinemia. II. Delayed hypersensitivity and homograft survived in a child with thymic alymphoplasia. Pediatrics 33:164, 1964

28. Kay HEM, Soothill JF: Transplanting the thymus. Lancet 1:571, 1969

29. Elves MW, Collinge M, Israëls MCG: The potential of lymphocytes from patients with leukemia and reticuloses to transform under the influence of phytohaemagglutinin. Acta Haematol (Basel) 37:100, 1967

30. Amiel JL, Sekiguchi M, Garattini S, Palma V: Etude de l'effet immunodépresseur des composés chimiques utilsés en chimiothérapie anticancéreuse. Europ J Cancer 3:47, 1967

31. Southam CM: The immunologic status of patients with nonlymphomatous cancer. Cancer Res 28:1433, 1968

32. Miller DG: The immunologic capability of patients with lymphoma. Cancer Res 28:1441, 1968

33. Schneider M: Effet des chemiothérapies cytostatiques sur une réaction d'hypersensibilité retardée. Rev Fr Etud Clin Biol 13:877, 1968

34. Migueres J, Jover A, Levy A: The effects on immune responses (tuberculin allergy and immune globulins) of treatment of inoperable lung cancer by antimitotic drugs. Poumon Coeur 243:351, 1968

35. Astaldi G, Airo R, Sauli S: In vitro studies on leukaemic cells, in Hayhoe's: Current Research in Leukaemia. Cambridge, New York, Cambridge Univ Pr, 1965, p 139

36. Trubowitz S, Masek B, Del Rosario A: Lymphocyte response to phytohemagglutinin in Hodgkin's disease, lymphatic leukemia and lymphosarcoma .Cancer 19:2019, 1966

37. Tansini G, Fornaroli E, Lusco G, Soresi E: Sull'immunità cellulare nei tumori solidi indagata mediante l'allergometria alla tubercolina e al BCG, e sue modificazioni per effetto di chemioterapici. Boll Ist Sieroter Milan 49:499, 1970

38. Miller JFAP, Osoba D: Current concepts of the immunological function of the thymus. Physiol Rev 47:437, 1967

AUTHOR INDEX

Amato, D., 54
Ammann, Arthur J., 61, 189

Benacerraf, Baruj, 129
Bergsagel, D.E., 54
Bockman, Dale E., 27
Buckner, C.D., 96, 103

Clarysse, A.M., 54
Clift, R.A., 96, 103
Cooper, Max D., 27
Cowan, D.H., 54

Dicke, K.A., 88
Di Paolo, Nicola, 223

Ellman, Leonard, 129

Fass, K.G., 103
Fefer, A., 96, 103
Funk, D.D., 96

Glucksberg, H., 96
Good, R.A., 61
Graw, R.G. Jr., 173
Green, Ira, 129
Greenwald, Harris L., 11

Hanna, M.G. Jr., 199
Hong, R., 61

Irad, 173
Iscove, N.N., 54

Kaplan, Michael S., 11
Katz, David H., 129
Kirkpatrick, C.H., 173

Lawlor, Glenn J. Jr., 11
Lawton, Alexander R., 27
Lerner, K.G., 103

Marcolongo, Roberto, 223
Marshall, W.H., 113
McCulloch, E.A., 54
Meuwissen, H.J., 61
Mickelson, E.M., 103
Mickenberg, 173
Miller, R.G., 54
Mitchison, N.A., 149

Neerhout, Robert C., 11
Neiman, P., 103

Paul, William E., 129
Perkins, Herbert, 189
Phillips, R.A., 54

Ragab, A.H., 54
Ramberg, R.E., 96
Rapp, Herbert J., 199
Rich, R.R., 173
Rogentine, G.N., 173
Rudolph, R., 103

Salmon, Sydney, 189
Santos, George W., 72
Schaefer, U.W., 88
Sengar, Dharmendra P.S., 11
Senn, J.S., 54
Smith, T.K., 173
Snodgrass, M.J., 199
Stiehm, E. Richard, 11
Storb, R., 96, 103

Terasaki, Paul I., 11
Thomas, E.D., 96, 103

van Bekkum, D.W., 88

Wara, Diane W., 189

Zbar, Berton, 199

KEY-WORD TITLE INDEX